REFERENCE

Havana

THE PORTRAIT OF A CITY

Other books by W. Adolphe Roberts

BIOGRAPHY:

Sir Henry Morgan: Buccaneer and Governor
Semmes of the Alabama

HISTORY:

The Caribbean: The Story of Our Sea of Destiny
The French in the West Indies
The U. S. Navy Fights
Lake Pontchartrain

TRAVEL:

Lands of the Inner Sea

NOVELS:

The Moralist
The Pomegranate
Royal Street
Brave Mardi Gras
Creole Dusk
The Single Star

VERSE:

Pierrot Wounded and Other Poems
Pan and Peacocks

Havana

THE PORTRAIT OF A CITY
by W. Adolphe Roberts

Coward-McCann, Inc.
New York

CONTENTS

PART I   **A Short History**

Sixteen pages of illustrations will be found following page 138.

Chapter 1

THERE ARE THREE HAVANAS

HAVANA is incomparably the chief city of the West Indies. The Caribbean region as a whole, comprising the coastal lands of the sea of that name and of the Gulf of Mexico, can offer only New Orleans as a rival, with Caracas as a runner-up. But in the archipelago Havana reigns: a city of over 700,000 with populous suburbs, a great commercial market, a focus of entertainment and the arts; in short, a capital in more than a national sense. Visitors from other Spanish-speaking units have long been attracted there, and with improved means of transportation English and French West Indians have started to come. The influx of pleasure seekers from the United States has swelled yearly, reaching a figure that makes Havana the principal tourist resort of the Western World. Nothing apparently can halt its growth.

It was not always in first place. Santo Domingo (now called Ciudad Trujillo) was the mother city of the Spanish Antilles. Santiago de Cuba was founded several years before Havana. Fantastic though this seems today, Port Royal, Jamaica, the haunt of the buccaneers, was a richer, more active port than Havana in the latter half of the seventeenth century and may have had a slightly larger population. But

Santiago was outstripped, Santo Domingo mouldered, and Port Royal went down in earthquake and flames.

The location of Havana is admirable, with its large deep-water harbor on one side, the open sea on the other, and the Morro heights opposite. Travelers always were impressed, whether they came by land or water, and now the view from the sky is one of far-flung beauty. But it takes imagination to chart clearly the development from earliest times. For a visitor to conceive of the town as an abstraction which expands vaguely around the spot where he finds himself at the moment is not enough. My object is to give him the portrait of a unique entity. Perhaps the best way to begin is to make the point that there are *three* Havanas, combined yet easily traceable as products of different historical periods. The entity turns out to be a triad.

They founded the city, after a couple of false starts, on what used to be described as a flat spur of land at the western side of the harbor mouth. The waterfront was later leveled out with filled ground. Narrow streets, some of them winding, were extended along the harbor and away from it, until in the middle of the seventeenth century it was decided to build walls with moats for the military protection of the community. The walls curved from the castle of La Punta on the sea, ran parallel to the street called *Monserrate* and connected with the harbor at the hospital of San Francisco de Paula. This fixed the borders of the original Havana, the city that was *intramuros*, or within the walls.

Settlements had already sprung up beyond. They grew with marked rapidity during the latter part of the eighteenth century and throughout the nineteenth century. Soon they had merged and become an important city, which was declared annexed in 1851. The new section begins at the Prado; the Hotel Nacional, on the site of the Santa Clara Battery, may be considered its limit on the ocean side.

Linked suburbs, starting with the Vedado and including Miramar and Marianao, extend along the sweep of the Gulf shore and bulge inland to absorb what used to be a scattering of villages. This is the third Havana, the most recent one, a child of the present century, which could not have developed on so grand a scale if it had not been for the automobile. With ancient means of transportation, only the Vedado—congested, smaller than it is today—could have been woven into the capital.

In noting characteristics, let us employ the simplest names: Old Havana, New Havana, and Suburban Havana. It should be remarked that Morro Castle, the Cabaña, and Casa Blanca on the other side of the harbor, are officially part of the city, but that contiguous Marianao to the west is a separate municipality.

The buildings of Old Havana (I do not speak here of modern replacements for business purposes) are nearly all of stone, adobe brick, rubble and mortar, or other forms of plaster construction. Fire hazards caused wood to be frowned upon at an early date; the Spanish settlers never fancied it, anyway. The structures stand tightly packed together, the front walls flush with the pavements, except for a few of the palaces and noble mansions which could afford precious space for arcades. Patios with gardens are numerous, however. Roofs are flat and balconies small.

The narrowness of the streets is partly due to the fact that such thoroughfares were easier to defend against attackers, partly to the ease with which they could be kept cool by stretching awnings above them. The original plan was for a closely united city which could be covered on foot and never in dreams would attain a population of more than a hundred thousand. It is studded with churches, convents, and surviving fortresses, the general effect being Mediterranean and in particular a modified southern Spanish. Cuban architects agree that Old Havana is not Andaluz, but it is without doubt a daughter of Sevilla, Córdoba, Málaga, and Cádiz. The tinting of walls in pastel shades, the prevailing color being a yellowish umber, enhances this effect.

New Havana also is Mediterranean Spanish in style, showing a gradual, normal evolution of taste. The streets are wider, more regularly laid out. A certain utilitarianism of apartment buildings and workshops, all looking pretty much alike, has replaced the serried, ornamental houses of days gone by. Not but what some very fine mansions were erected in New Havana, especially on the Prado and other open reaches. Some of these have doorways through which carriages were driven, great patios beyond, and balconies of wrought ironwork both on the street and the patio. There was elbow-room outside the walls—*extramuros*—and the rich made full use of it. The generality created a quarter that would have been like comparable middle-class quarters in Europe if it had not been for the tall palms and the blaze of tropical flowers. None of the centers of colonial administration stood here. Enthusiasm for building churches had fallen off; the emphasis was on convent hospitals and schools. The university is on the western edge of the district, and adjoining it the Quinta de los Molinos, summer residence of the governors of Cuba. Príncipe Castle, close to this point, and Atarés Castle, to the eastward at the head of the harbor, complete the ring of the city's defences.

Suburban Havana is an utterly different manifestation. It abandons the old romance, and from the architectural standpoint has plainly been more influenced by North America than Spain. The homes are surrounded by gardens, wherever possible. Many are on a magnificent scale, suggestive of the palaces of millionaires in California. The tropical setting adds a good deal to the rows and rows of flats such as one might see in Los Angeles or Miami. Country clubs flourish, featuring outdoor sports for both sexes. The Casino Nacional with its beautiful grounds has to meet competition from race tracks and baseball parks. Broad landscaped avenues are like river beds along which rush endless streams of cars. Motor boats dart in and out of the havens of aquatic clubs on the shimmering blue of the Gulf of Mexico.

Yet the three Havanas are locked together as one. Among the connecting links we find the bizarre detail of extremely modernistic buildings, which appear here and there without regard to the age or width of the streets where they stand. They look like signatures not of a period but of a fad. A little research will show evidence of other, earlier fads, which although less glaring were probably thought outlandish at first sight. The charm of the city is great enough to permit it to spare room for such curios, as a plain town in the United States, for example, is not able to do.

Dream backward in time and consider what the scene must have looked like to the founders of Havana. They pre-empted their little flat cape which was situated so conveniently at the entrance of a fine harbor. But the surrounding country was no sandy, infertile level such as would have faced them in near by Florida or the Bahamas. This Cuban territory of theirs was lush and rolling. Immediately behind the settlement stood a small hill, later called the Loma de Peña Pobre, or the Loma del Angel from the church built there. Larger hills rose farther out, a wide succession of them: the hill which was to be the site of the university, Príncipe, Atarés, the Loma del Burro. A stream named the Luyanó emptied itself into the bay, and a few miles to the west the important Almendares River joined the sea.

Grassy savannas alternated with dense growths of forest. It was land rich enough to create commerce for a respectable little port.

A settler could have climbed to his rooftop and taken in most of this panorama with a circular glance. He would have laughed indulgently, as at a fairy story, if told that the land his eyes could reach—all of it, with more beyond —would in four hundred years have been built upon and become part of his city of Havana.

Chapter 2

THE FOUNDING OF THE CITY

Two false starts were made before Havana was actually founded. Diego Velásquez, the conqueror of Cuba, who came across from Hispaniola in 1511, established seven cities in the next four years. The last and most westerly of these received the name of San Cristóbal de la Habana, but it was on the shallow bay of Batabanó near the modern town of that name on the south coast. Pánfilo de Narváez chose the site, and Velásquez visited and approved of it. A curse of bad luck seemed to rest on everything done by Narváez, that tall red-haired adventurer, whose voice is described as sounding with a hollow boom as though he were speaking under a vault, and who reveled in killing Indians. Batabanó was lovely with its coral gardens visible below the surface of iridescent water; it could never be a practical harbor for ships of deep draught. Nothing is known about this original Havana, except that it was the last point of call in Cuba for Hernando Cortés before his departure for Mexico.

The discontented settlers were already planning to move. It was remembered that in 1508 Sebastián de Ocampo had circumnavigated Cuba for the first time and had reported the existence of a fine port on the north coast where he had careened his ships, the longitude being the same as that of Batabanó. Explorers now rediscovered it. They were tempted by the Almendares River, told their fellow townsmen that its mouth was the ideal spot on account of the water supply, and accordingly an attempt was made to build the town there. The location proved to be far too open to the sea, and at some date toward the end of 1519 the final shift occurred.

The origin of the name is obscure. Some authorities hold that it was a corruption of Savanna; others point out that there was once a north-European port called *Havanna*, deriving from the Anglo-Saxon word "haven." But there exists a letter by Velásquez in which he comments that that part of Cuba was governed by the cacique, Habaguanex, and it is reasonable to suppose that Spanish garbling of a native title produced *La Habana*. It should not be forgotten that when "b" or "v" occur between vowels they are pronounced alike in the Castilian tongue, the sound being a sort of combination of the two letters.

Siboney Indians lived thereabouts, as Velásquez makes clear, but they were not numerous or hostile and they escaped the worst forms of cruelty practiced on their fellows at the eastern end of the island. The Spaniards enslaved some of them as domestic servants and workmen, ignoring them otherwise in the founding of the city. Precisely what was done at the start, however, on the flat cape opposite the Morro headland will never be known. All official records prior to 1550 were destroyed, probably in one of the raids by corsairs which occurred frequently from 1537 onward.

There is the tradition that the adoption of the site was celebrated on November 16th, St. Christopher's Day, by a mass said in the shade of a giant ceiba or silk-cotton tree at the northeastern edge of the present Plaza de Armas. A shrine called the Templete has been erected there. It contains a bust of Christopher Columbus, and in front of it stands a ceiba popularly believed to have been grown from a cutting of the ancient tree when the latter was dying of old age. The story is myth, pure and simple. We have no documents to prove that a mass was said in the open air at that spot or anywhere else, though it is very likely that a religious ceremony of some sort took place.

Spanish colonial cities were built according to a pattern prescribed by the Council of the Indies. There must be a central plaza on which faced the church, the governor's residence and other official edifices. The streets must be laid out from this at right angles and as straightly as possible. It is obvious that the plan was followed in Havana. The first church was on the Plaza de Armas, the cathedral being of much later construction. The first street of commercial prominence was Oficios, running eastward from the plaza and parallel with the waterfront.

Primitive indeed were the buildings, not much better than the *bohíos* or thatched huts of the Indians. Even the church was of wattle and mud, with a thatched roof. As soon as possible, flimsy walls were replaced by *mampostería* (broken stone and sand enclosed in plaster) and tiled roofs were gradually introduced. The so-called "Fisherman's Hut," complete with adjoining pump and trough, the oldest complete dwelling to be seen in Havana today, is in the patio of the Santa Clara Convent, now occupied by the Department of Public Works. It dates at least seventy-five years from the founding of the city.

Santiago was the capital of Cuba, but Havana took on almost immediate importance as a result of the conquest of Mexico. It lay on the shortest route between Veracruz and Spain. Ships going in either direction would naturally call there for supplies, take refuge in the harbor if threatened by an enemy, or use it as a rallying point for expeditions. Velásquez, the first governor, clung to Santiago but appointed a *teniente a guerra*, or special aide, to represent him in Havana. For twenty-five years subsequent governors divided their time between Santiago and Havana, while the Crown in its dilatory way refused to admit that the new town was becoming the real center of Cuba's activities. On the broader stage of the Antilles, it played the role in the west that Santo Domingo still played in the middle.

As early as 1521 an illustrious name was connected with Havana when Juan Ponce de León came there, mortally wounded, from Florida where he had been hunting for the fountain of youth. Pedro de Alvarado and other lieutenants of Cortés paid visits on their leader's business. In 1523 a treasure fleet carrying gold, jewels, and feathered Aztec cloaks touched at Havana on its way to Europe; French privateers cut out two of the galleons near the Azores, and the booty stirred the envy of the court in Paris. This event led before long to the forming of convoys which assembled at Havana for the perilous run across the Atlantic.

It is clear that the pioneer residents were traders on a fairly large scale. Apart from the business done by the ship chandlers, hides were the chief native product exported. We are told by chroniclers that the community was excessively lawless and addicted to gambling. Cards and dice were played with much brawling in all the taverns and various private houses. The streets were unlighted, and those who went about after dark risked assault with cudgel and dagger. There was a shortage of women, yet enough of them for harlotry to flourish. Syphilis was rife, an importation from Spain, for the old belief that this was a New World disease that infected Europe is demonstrably false. The Siboney Indians suffered from a mild venereal malady which they cured easily with infusions from the green wood of the *guayacán* tree, called in English "lignum vitae."

Fledgling Havana rated as one of the most sinful towns in America. A place of the sort, still unfortified, was bound to attract the attention of foreign marauders. French pirates were the first to challenge the dictum of Pope Alexander VI, giving Spain the entire region, which the latter had declared to be a closed preserve. They appeared in 1537 and 1538, raiding throughout the Caribbean and attacking Havana in both years. The 1537 affair was spectacular. A single Frenchman drove the shipping to cover off Havana, coolly entered the harbor and for three hours surveyed the vessels lying there. He then sailed down the coast westward toward Mariel. Pursued by three Spanish sail, he turned upon them, burned two and captured the third. Accounts differ as to whether this pirate came back and sacked Havana. But the one who arrived the following year seized the town, occupied it for fifteen days, used the torch freely and did a thorough job of pillaging. When he left he took even the church bells with him.

These coups left the primitive settlement virtually in ashes. In the rebuilding, which was pushed with energy, wood and thatch were discarded as much as possible in favor of stone. A rough fort was erected to the west of the plaza. The developments overlapped the intervention in Cuban affairs—with Cuba merely a means to an end—of the glowing, romantic figure of Hernando de Soto.

Soto was an hidalgo who had gone with Pizarro to Peru and had there done two legendary things. He had personally laid hands on Atahualpa, the Inca monarch, and dragged him into the incredible slavery that had ended only with his murder. Soto had also discovered the mountain pass that led to Cuzco the magnificent, thus becoming the guide to one of the looting orgies of all time and obtaining a considerable share of the treasure for himself. He had returned to Spain worth more than a hundred thousand ducats, had married the great lady and beauty, Isabel de Bobadilla. But he was a man of quenchless ambition. He wanted to be the discoverer of his own Indian empire. The luckless Narváez had gone to Florida to look for one and had perished, but four survivors of his expedition had reached Mexico on foot after crossing an immense territory. The stories told enflamed the imagination of Hernando de Soto, who got the king to appoint him governor of Cuba and *adelantado* or military administrator of Florida.

Cuba was needed by Soto as headquarters. The name "Florida" he interpreted as signifying all of the North American continent which had not yet been explored. His commission allowed him the boon of equipping forces at his own expense for a foray into the unknown. He landed with great fanfare at Santiago de Cuba in the summer of 1538, accompanied by his wife, about a thousand armed men, priests and volunteers of all descriptions. The old capital staged a fiesta in his honor, with bullfights and dancing. But a few weeks after he had taken over the government he sent the ships with his household establishment and most of the troops to Havana, while he paraded through the island escorted by knights and squires.

His impact on the reviving port was sensational. Its permanent inhabitants were exceeded in number by Hernando de Soto's soldiery and the camp followers attracted to him in Cuba. Havana found itself over-run by the newcomers. They were compelled to go to work and build houses for their own shelter, and in consequence the size of the town was much increased. Soto revised the defensive system and took personal charge of the completion of the fort. The lavish preparation for his venture to Florida started more than one mercantile firm on the road to fortune.

He sent two advance parties to the peninsula to find the best landing place. Their reports were marked by gloom, but Soto would not allow anything to discourage him. He sailed at full strength in May, 1539, after formally appointing his wife Doña Isabel to act as governor of Cuba in his absence. His terrible hardships, his discovery of the Mississippi only to die and be buried in its waters, make one of the most tragic stories in the annals of the conquistadors. Five years passed before a remnant of his force escaped to Mexico and told what had happened.

Tradition has it that Doña Isabel died of grief, after having spent all of her leisure during the five years watching from her apartments in the tower of the fort for the return of Soto. Her vigil could not have been kept from the existing Fuerza, though guides persist in saying that it was. La Fuerza replaced the Soto fort, as will be noted in due course. Nor did Doña Isabel weep herself to death on learning of her husband's fate. The chronicles prove that she signed documents as a very old woman in Spain.

The collapse of Soto's dreamful project reacted harmfully upon Havana. Gay swaggerers who had equipped themselves without stint and were to have brought back untold treasure—where were they? Where was the boom of yesterday? The citizens were thankful that they had had the strength to repulse a French pirate who came with four small ships in 1543, and the following year the worst was known. Doña Isabel probably had something to do with the appointment of the next governor, who was a relation of hers, a young lawyer named Juanés Dávila. Florida, abandoned for the time being, was not included in his charge.

This man and his two successors, also lawyers, behaved curiously to say the least. Dávila took office in Santiago, as required by law, but in a few months he married a rich old widow of that town and trumped up reasons for shifting his household to Havana. There he practiced graft in so shameless a manner that he was removed from office. A search revealing gold bars buried in the dirt floor of one of his holdings, he was thereupon sent to Spain for trial. His wife's money was used to buy him out of trouble, and he returned to Cuba to become a flourishing merchant.

Antonio de Chávez, who succeeded Dávila, followed a similar course. When indicted for dishonesty, he was accused in addition of plotting to transfer the seat of government to Havana, and of "corrupting the women of the island"—a large order surely. He spent several years in prison, then received permission to leave Spain for Peru where he did well.

Dr. Gonzalo Pérez de Angulo, the last of the trio, conducted himself more prudently at first and lasted longer. Instead of seeking to make Havana the capital, he simply moved there quietly in 1550 and established a precedent which others followed. He made efforts to improve the administration while lining his own pockets. If he had not had to face the supreme assault of freebooters on Havana, he might have been thought a capable governor.

Chapter 3

THE LUTHERAN TRAVESTY

IN JULY, 1555, there were fifty-one resident citizens of Havana, of whom thirty-eight were landowning heads of families. Their women and minor children may be estimated at 300. About 125 free Indian servants lived in the city, and the number of Indian and Negro slaves ran between 200 and 300. A few priests were attached to the single church. Sailors and other transients were always present, but it would be an exaggeration to assume a total count of 1,000. Among the outstanding family names were Rojas, Ynestrosa, and Calderon. The two most significant men next to the governor and more important than he in the long run were Juan de Rojas, owner of the finest house, and Juan de Lobera, warden of the fort, who had married a Rojas.

The church was a stone building nearing completion; it replaced the original shoddy structure and stood on part of the site of the present municipal palace. Lobera had personally, with great energy, strengthened the fort of Hernando de Soto's time. He had gone to Spain and induced the authorities to give him two fairly large cannon and two falconets with a supply of ammunition. A short distance eastward, in full view of the fort, was Juan de Rojas's big stone house. The governor lived in an inferior residence on the Plaza de Armas. The farther reaches of the town had no defensive system against an enemy who might achieve a landing.

War had broken out once more between Spain and France in 1552. Tired of leaving mere pirates to benefit from raids in the Caribbean, the French king commissioned two well-known captains as privateers to do what damage they could and bring back their plunder for division between themselves and the Crown. These men were François le Clerc, called *Pié de Palo* by the Spaniards on account of his peg-leg; and Jacques de Sores, a Protestant by religion. They shared the field, after having made demonstrations in force at Santo Domingo, Cartagena and Nombre de Dios. Le Clerc took Hispaniola and Puerto Rico, while Sores was assigned Cuba.

Such enterprises developed slowly in the sixteenth century. The year 1554 was well advanced before Sores passed from lesser feats to the sacking of Santiago de Cuba, where he collected 80,000 pesos. When rumors of this event were confirmed Havana began to worry, without taking protective steps of any consequence, let it be said. Lookouts were posted on the Morro heights across the harbor, and two mounted sentries patrolled the coast on both sides of the mouth of the Almendares River.

Early in the morning of July 10, 1555, the Morro reported a brigantine cruising westward. The cannon-signal agreed upon was fired. Twelve picked men hurried to the fort and placed themselves at the disposal of the warden, Lobera. The governor appeared in the Plaza with a small escort. Presently the mounted guards came galloping into the city and announced that the mysterious ship was French, that it had dropped anchor in a cove at the point where the San Lázaro tower is now to be seen in the Parque

Maceo, and that a large force of heavily armed men was being disembarked. Jacques de Sores had arrived.

The total Spanish force available was a militia of sixteen men with horses, and sixty-five afoot. A little more than half of these were land-owning citizens, while the rest were artisans, clerks, sailors, servants, and various persons of mixed blood. If a resolute, united stand had been made, the French might have been driven back. But as soon as Governor Angulo was fully informed he fled the city with his family, accompanied by a considerable number of his armed neighbors. This party circled the bay and struck inland a few miles to Guanabacoa, a village which had been established as a sort of reservation for free aboriginal Indians.

Lobera furiously resented the cowardly behavior of the governor. He announced that he would do his utmost to hold the fort, and after he had admitted refugees of both sexes he found himself with a fighting force of thirty. Four men used crossbows. The rest had harquebuses, but there was a shortage of gunpowder both for the cannon and the small arms. The food supplies in the fort might be rationed to last for ten days.

The French marched in good order through the woods that came down to the seashore. They entered the community without opposition, at once seized the Rojas stone house as a headquarters, invested the fort and demanded its surrender. Lobera contemptuously refused. He opened fire with his guns, prevented the brigantine from entering the harbor and also drove off a second ship that had put in an appearance. Toward evening a ball shot away the privateers' flag, which had been hoisted over the Rojas house. Meanwhile three attacks on the fort were repulsed, though the gates were set afire and the flames spread to the wooden tower. Lobera had his bugles blown all night and ordered the biggest gun to be discharged at intervals, hoping that this would shame Governor Angulo into counterattacking. But at dawn the ammunition was almost exhausted and there was no sign of reinforcements.

We have no reliable information on the numbers of the French. At least a hundred must have been ranged for a final assault, and others were landing. They terrified the aged and the women and children, who fell on their knees before Lobera and begged him to make terms. He decided to capitulate on receiving a promise from Sores that there would be no raping or butchery. The male Spaniards of military age were held in the Rojas house and the noncombatants sent to their homes.

Captain Jacques de Sores had assuredly not behaved as a cutthroat or blackguard up to that point. He may be assumed to have had a poor opinion of Catholics, but he regarded himself as a loyal Frenchman on the king's business, and if it seems strange to us that a Catholic monarch of those days should have commissioned a Protestant we must remember that the Wars of Religion had not yet started in France. Sores belonged to the sect of Calvinists known as Huguenots, and he had enlisted crews of the same faith. To the Spaniards he was a Lutheran, for they applied that term to all Protestants.

He set the ransom of Havana at 30,000 pesos and one hundred loads of cassava bread, remarking that he was treating the town generously in comparison with Santiago which had paid him 80,000 pesos. The residents vowed they would be able to pay only about a third of the sum asked. Sores flew into a passion, but agreed to a truce while ways and means were being considered. Looting by individual privateers was held to a minimum. Whether Angulo was notified and approved the truce is not clear. The governor, however, raised a force of ninety-five armed Spaniards, nine of whom were mounted, as well as eighty Siboneys and more than

two hundred Negroes carrying sticks and stones. The entire
district as far east as Matanzas was drawn upon. A week
after the surrender of the city Angulo staged a night march
from Guanabacoa and had almost reached the Rojas house
before he was detected.

Some of the French had been sleeping outside the fort
and other strong points. They suffered losses, a brother of
Sores being among the killed. The rest dashed to shelter and
a fight raged at dawn. Captain de Sores in the Rojas house
was infuriated at what he held to be a treacherous breach
of the truce. He ordered his prisoners put to death, and
some twenty-five were slain. Then he went to the private
room where Lobera was confined, intending to kill him with
his own hand. Lobera stood up to him. Sores ended by
praising the warden as the only brave, honorable Spaniard
in Havana and sparing him against a personal ransom of
2,200 pesos—a sum that eventually was paid.

During the course of the morning, Angulo was defeated
and driven back to the countryside. Sores harshly demanded
his levy of treasure and food, and on hearing that only
what he called a "miserable 1,000 pesos" had been collected
he let loose his men on Havana. The place, he declared, was
to be relentlessly pillaged and then destroyed.

What followed was no ordinary sacking of a town. The
robbery was thorough, the devastation complete. All the
buildings and all the craft in the harbor had the torch put
to them. Most houses were burned to the ground. Those
of stone construction were gutted, the Rojas house coming
off best. Nearby plantations were visited and the homes
demolished. But the unique feature was the flaring of latent
religious fanaticism. It did not take the form of massacre.
The privateers ran wild over the chance to insult the Catholic faith in every possible manner, and they wanted a living
populace to see what they were doing.

They plundered the church, desecrated it with sacrilegious miming and the spattering of ordure, dragged the images outdoors and kicked them around. They burned the building, which was left with nothing but its exterior walls standing. The priests, of course, were made to undergo every conceivable affront. Privateers costumed themselves in vestments and altar cloths, stuck the sacred images on poles and paraded through the ruins of Havana, roaring with laughter, halting at intervals to stab madonna or saint with bloody poniards. There was a chapel at the hospital. This also was polluted and the structure burned.

Sores relished the show and cheered on his hearties. He could scarcely have dreamed that the episode was to have an effect upon the history of the Caribbean. The Spaniards called it the Lutheran Travesty. They never forgot or forgave it. Two hundred years of reprisals in the New World on the score of sect and creed may be said to have started on that day.

On August 5th, or twenty-six days after his landing, Captain de Sores departed with his ships and his booty. He had waited for favoring winds, a calm sea. He got them and brilliant moonlight too, as the official report carried by Lobera to Spain attested mournfully. "Our Lord knows what He does," it ran, "when to a Lutheran like that one [Sores, whose crimes are recapitulated] He gives victory in everything and good weather by which to navigate. His Divine Majesty knows what He does and why He does it."

Lesser French privateers paid two visits before the end of October, but they obtained little for their pains. A period with a curse upon it had drawn to a close.

So Havana set to work to rebuild for the second time. Confirmation of its destiny showed plainly in the speed with which a greater number of homes were erected than had been there before. The decline that had followed Hernando de Soto's misadventure was reversed. New citizens arrived from the four quarters of the Spanish domain. True, they were described as a profligate, violent lot, including merchants who had failed elsewhere, deserters from ships, unfrocked clerics and women who had run away from their husbands. All were gamblers, in one sense or another. But their eagerness to settle at this spot, while the tendency elsewhere in the Caribbean was to desert the islands for the mainland, proved their faith in the future of the port. They guessed astutely.

If such pleasantries as knifing the man to whom you had lost at cards, or poisoning a concubine to make place for a fresh one, were common—the chroniclers say they were—it was merely in character with other young and bloodsplashed ports of the region.

Chapter 4
KEY OF THE NEW WORLD

PÉREZ DE ANGULO had been charged with irregularities in office before the assault by Sores, and it had been decided to replace him as governor. He had not redeemed himself during the fighting, in fact had made everyone doubly eager to be rid of him. The unpredictable delays of those times left him at the head of things until March of the next year while his successor-designate, Diego de Mazariegos, wrestled with the hardships of red tape and ship-wreck. Angulo was most averse to leaving Havana, and as will be seen he never did.

Mazariegos had obviously better qualifications than the three lawyers who had preceded him. He was a soldier who had been with Cortés in Mexico, had fought Indians else-where, and had shown talent as a military administrator. Havana needed to be fortified as well as rebuilt. Its population needed to be ruled firmly. Mazariegos proved himself the man for the job, and he lasted almost ten years.

There loomed behind and over him, to be sure, the portentous figure of Admiral Pedro Menéndez de Avilés, Spain's leading colonial strategist of the period, who had begun as a commander of convoys from Mexico and who ended as captain general of the armada "to guard the coasts and ports of the Indies." Menéndez drew plans for the construction of impregnable castles at all the key points of the region, including Havana, Veracruz, and Cartagena. It was Menéndez who later retaliated for the Lutheran Travesty by wiping out the French Huguenot colony at the mouth of the St. John's River, Florida, and founding St. Augustine instead, the oldest city in what is now the United States.

But our subject is Havana. The lesser works that strengthened the port were started under Mazariegos and he made it possible for the engineers sent from Spain to push some of them through to completion. A tall white watchtower on the site of the Morro was wholly his project. It was replaced soon by the mighty castle. In the city itself arose the first walls that we may still see there, and of these the most important was La Fuerza. The clearing of the ground on which it was to be constructed swept away outbuildings of the old fort where Doña Isabel had kept vigil for her husband and which Lobera had defended, the Rojas house, and several other masonry homes of leading citizens.

We shrug our shoulders in amazement at the dilatory methods of the age when we learn that the razing was not done
until 1558, three years after the visit of the privateers, and
that La Fuerza was not approximately ready until 1573. The
guns could have been served from partly finished bastions,
no doubt. This did not have to be tested, due to luck and
the naval precautions of Admiral Menéndez.

On the executive side, Mazariegos had a deal of trouble
with the Havanese. He appears to have enjoyed it. The man
was a curious mixture of disciplinarian, official moralist, and
personal free-liver. He was severe with crimes of violence,
sparing no one, however highly placed. He seized a whip
and flogged one of his own nephews, accusing him among
other things of "lechery." Yet Mazariegos had without the
least concealment taken as his mistress Francisca, a daughter of ex-Governor Angulo, and had laughed at the protests
of her mother and the clergy. Angulo could have had no
objections, for he and Mazariegos were close friends until
the former's death toward the end of the year. Eventually,
under pressure, Mazariegos married the lady, remarking that
he had always considered her as being his wife in the eyes
of God. He got even by casting doubt upon the chastity of
the bishop of Cuba.

This disdainful treatment of the representatives of the
Church can be accounted for by the fact, which every historian has noted, that Cuba was less devout than other
Spanish colonies. It is difficult to say why it should have
been so. The lusty adventurers who conquered nearby Mexico professed extreme piety and dowered the Church heavily from the start. Those who settled in Cuba, and especially
Havana, took no such stand. We find that the parish church
looted by Sores and burned to its four walls was about the
last public building restored under Mazariegos. For five
years, from 1555 to 1560, there was no consecrated place of

worship in Havana. Mass was said at different makeshift altars. The Cabildo, or municipal council, often expressed its antipathy for friars in general. As for the bishop, his cathedral was in Santiago and one did not see much of him.

All the early governors need not be discussed. Among them was Menéndez himself, who served for five years though retaining his post of captain general of the fleets and usually represented in the island by a lieutenant. Menéndez, incidentally, was a very religious man, even a bigot. But his two immediate successors, Montalvo and Carreño, leaned so far in the opposite direction that they were both excommunicated by the bishop. Don Francisco Carreño uttered a quip on the matter that has been widely quoted. "And this is no country in which to pass a single night excommunicated," he said when the news was brought to him. He was not thinking of the peril to his soul, but of his enemies who would know that a man cut off from communion with the Church could be killed by anyone without penalty.

The next governor but one after Carreño was also appointed captain general of Cuba, so as to give him equality with high-ranking military and naval commanders whose duties brought them to Havana. The custom was perpetuated. Though addressed formally by both titles, the chief executive came to be described in ordinary talk as the captain-general.

In 1585 Sir Francis Drake led twenty-five ships carrying 2,300 men to the Caribbean, this being the most formidable fleet of privateers to date. He captured and plundered Santo Domingo. Early in 1586 he performed the much greater exploit of taking Cartagena by storm. It was his intention to attack Havana on his return voyage to England, but when he arrived at the end of May he only made a demonstration at the mouth of the harbor. La Fuerza looked like a tough nut, and he did not care to risk losing the treasure already aboard his ships. Instead he proceeded to St. Augustine, Florida, which he destroyed, and to Roanoke Island, North Carolina, where he rescued the survivors of an ill-fated colony founded there by Sir Walter Raleigh.

Drake was of all privateer captains the one who had most impressed the Spanish colonial empire. He had become a half-legendary being, *El Drake*, a name translated by some as "The Dragon," since both Drake and dragon are from the Latin *draco*. But the Spaniards have the same spelling for dragon that we do. The *Drake*, pronounced in two syllables, was a new species of monster who made terrible threats and actually carried them out. That he had looked at Havana was warning enough. So in spite of the staggering bill that Philip II had to meet two years later as a result of the rout of the Invincible Armada, with Drake as second in command on the English side, the monarch agreed to spend still another fortune to put Havana beyond danger of capture by the navies of the period.

A famous engineer named Antonelli arrived in 1589 and studied the problem. The conclusion he reached was the inevitable minimum. There must be a fortress of the first order on the Morro heights and a lesser one on the point immediately opposite. This would make La Fuerza a mere secondary post within the harbor. Of course there should have been a city wall, and the Cabaña ridge, Atarés, and Príncipe should all have been fortified; for without these a land attack would remain possible. But the Morro and the Punta represented the utmost that the regime could undertake. They were usable in eight years, a miracle of speed when we recall how long the smaller Fuerza had taken to build, though the Morro was not declared completed until 1630.

With the coming of Antonelli and a new governor, Havana was proclaimed by royal edict in 1589 the capital of Cuba in place of Santiago. Five years afterward it was created a city. The proud Cabildo adopted a coat of arms showing three castles—Fuerza, Morro, and Punta—beneath which was a golden key. The following civic motto was devised: "Key of the New World and Bulwark of the Western Indies." Various ornaments in connection with the coat of arms were used from time to time. Prints are to be seen enclosed by the collar of the Golden Fleece, which was quite unjustified. The castles and the key remained fixed. This design and the use of the motto were confirmed by the Crown about fifty years afterward.

The symbols of the key and the bulwark were far from being bombast. Havana's location between the Gulf of Mexico and the Florida Strait was the most commanding in the Antilles, particularly because Cuba was so long an island that it shut off any approach to the Caribbean from the Atlantic Ocean for 700 miles. Where Mexico was concerned, Havana had become vital, for the continental viceroyalty had no good ports of its own on the Gulf. Veracruz, the best one, was protected so raggedly by islets that it was called the "pocket full of holes." Mexico, ordered by Spain to provide some of the funds for the building of the Morro and Punta, responded gladly. We shall find emphasis on this relationship growing stronger and stronger. It even came to be said that Havana was the naval port of Mexico.

Commerce, which had made an excellent start because of the needs of Mexico, was not allowed to develop naturally. Spain had adopted the strictest form of mercantilism, or the closed economy, in her dealings with her colonies. All trading had to be done through specified ports in the Peninsula, and this was interpreted to prevent the colonies even from having direct traffic with one another. Every order had to be handled by a merchant in Spain, as middleman. Cuba might not sell hides to Panama, for example. If hides were wanted in Panama the proper authorities were informed, and the goods would make a round trip—at greatly enhanced prices—from Cuba to the Isthmus, via Spain.

The cultivation of the vine was prohibited in the New World by statute in 1595, so as to leave no choice but to purchase Spanish wine or go without. Any form of manufacturing which could compete with an industry in Spain was prohibited. Taxes of every description, including a 10 per cent sales tax, made anything bought in a colonial shop from three to ten times more expensive than it was in Spain. Such was the state of affairs at the end of the sixteenth century. The policy would become increasingly rigid for the next hundred and fifty years. Though this bottling up harmed Havana, the city met some of its requirements by the practice of smuggling on a large scale. It was counted one of the most rebellious of Spanish American ports.

Houses in 1600 were seldom higher than one story. All those of any pretensions were of *mampostería* masonry, the walls often two feet thick for security and coolness. Cellars were unknown because of the miry soil befouled with sewage. Flat roofs prevailed. One high, broad doorway connected with the street, admitting to the courtyard the owner's vehicles if he had any. The windows were tall, heavily guarded by iron bars, destitute of glass but with wooden shutters behind the bars.

All curving lanes from the early times had been straightened. The widest street was only twenty-two feet from housefront to housefront. Sidewalks ranged between one and a half feet and three and a half feet in width. A little paving with stone blocks had been done, but many street crossings were mudholes that had to be bridged with planks. There was no public system of lighting the streets at night.

As the century closed the Franciscan Order completed a fine church and monastery on the waterfront, dedicated naturally to San Francisco. It was so radically reconstructed in 1737 that the building we know today as the home of the ministry of communications must be ascribed to the eighteenth century. In 1599 the first theatrical performance in Havana's history was given at the military barracks.

Chapter 5

IN THE SHADOW OF THE BUCCANEERS

NOTHING MUCH happened in Havana during the seventeenth century. This bald statement occurs in book after book. Imagine, a city that had eighty years of turbulent life behind it is said to have spent the next three generations uneventfully. Things of great moment to the inhabitants took place, of course, between 1601 and 1700, but historical research workers have neglected them because the obviously melodramatic did indeed pass Havana by. This, for instance, was the century of the buccaneers. They menaced the Key of the Western World more than once— and stayed their hands. The maritime powers of northern Europe started to establish permanent colonies in the Caribbean. They caused terror by extending their operations to Santiago de Cuba and other strong points, but left Havana alone. Immunity was largely due to the prestige of Morro Castle, which had been built against Drake and which thwarted Morgan. Enough brewed in the offing to stir plenty of emotion.

Let us consider.

The first twenty-five years were preternaturally calm. Then the Dutch, who had lately shaken themselves free of Spanish oppression in the Netherlands, sent imposing forces to the New World under the auspices of their West India Company. Bowdoin Hendriks, the burgomaster of Edam, sacked San Juan, Puerto Rico, in 1625. He was followed by two famous admirals, Pieter Pieterszoon Heyn with thirty-one vessels, and Pieter Adriaanzoon Ita with twelve. Heyn was a national hero, who had twice in his youth been condemned to the galleys by the Spaniards, the first time with his own father as benchmate. The pair, Heyn in supreme command, were off Havana late in August, 1628. Thirty of their ships were present and 3,000 men, a huge expedition for the times. They feinted cautiously. When the Morro and the Punta fired against them, they pretended to be discouraged and retired to a distance of several miles. Their real object was to waylay the treasure fleet from Veracruz.

Cutting out galleons was an old story. Every great privateer had dreamed of ravishing a whole fleet. Drake had longed for one in vain. Now it was to be accomplished, and Havana had a grandstand seat for the terrifying show. The Spanish admiral, Juan de Benavides, allowed himself to be outmaneuvered. Instead of advancing into the wind that was blowing from the west, Heyn withdrew in the direction of Matanzas. When the plate fleet had been carried around the curve of Cuba by the Gulf Stream and the following wind, Heyn struck it behind its center and ran along with it, fighting masterfully. He captured nine ships at sea. Eight others tried to reach safety in Havana harbor, but he intercepted them and herded them on to the beaches within the bay of Matanzas and just outside it.

Booty said to be worth 15 million guilders was taken. When Heyn arrived with it in Rotterdam, Holland made him her chief admiral. That year the Dutch West India Company declared a 50 per cent dividend. The coup had been one of the most profitable in the history of Caribbean adventure.

The next attempt of the Dutch thereabouts was anti-climax. Cornelius Jols came in 1638 with twenty vessels, threatened the city harmlessly and then lurked down the coast, hoping to repeat the exploit of Heyn and Ita. A small convoy of seven galleons appeared, and Jols dashed confidently to take possession of them. But Carlos Ibarra, the Spanish commander, was no Benavides; he gave prompt and successful battle, capturing three Dutch ships and putting the rest to flight. Jols suffered a loss of 400 men.

Meanwhile the phenomenon of the buccaneers had been taking form. These unique freebooters were outlaws of all nationalities except the Spanish—deserters from armed forces, fugitives from religious persecution, escaped criminals or bondsmen—who tried at first to establish settlements in the neglected western half of Hispaniola. They lived chiefly off the herds of cattle and hogs that had been allowed to run wild, smoking the meat by a special process and building up a trade in it with passing ships. The Arawak name for this sort of smoked meat had been *boucan*, so they became *boucaniers*, or in English, buccaneers. The Spaniards dispersed them in the 1620's. They retired to certain strongholds, notably the small rockbound island of Tortuga, built craft of their own and took to the sea as robbers. The commands tended to group themselves according to their country of origin, and they boasted of the policy (not always kept) of sparing ships and towns that flew their old flag. Only the Spaniard was the enemy of all. This raised the buccaneers above the level of outright piracy.

Their success was extraordinary. They soon had scores of ships, many of which had been taken in battle. They were self-appointed privateers. Since they had no interests outside the Caribbean, they turned their victories and the plunder they obtained to local account. Thus they helped to shape the history of the region. The English, French, and Dutch authorities often gave them letters of marque during the wars with Spain and eventually succeeded in merging them with the different colonial systems.

In 1640 the buccaneers formed the Confederacy of the Brethren of the Coast. Until then their naval exploits had been more or less erratic and dependent on the ideas of individual captains. They now adopted a reasonably strict discipline and elected a supreme leader. Their first important admiral was Edward Mansvelt, who said he was a Dutchman from Curaçao, though some insisted that he was English and his real name Mansfield. Their second and far more effective admiral was Henry Morgan the Welshman.

Havana lived in constant dread of the buccaneers. But they did not appear so far to the north and west until after 1655, when Jamaica was lost by Spain, and the English among the marauders had made Port Royal their headquarters, leaving Tortuga to the French. The 1660's were to prove the banner decade of the "sweet trade," as its practitioners affectionately called it.

Jean David Nau, alias l'Ollonais, had his interest aroused by Havana in 1660. He was from the Sables d'Olonne on the Bay of Biscay, hence his *nom de guerre*. The chroniclers agree that he was probably the most sadistically cruel captain that the business ever knew. He personally beheaded prisoners, and he licked the blade after each stroke. He once gnawed at a heart he had just torn from a victim's breast. L'Ollonais, operating out of Tortuga, ran into bad luck on the Yucatan coast. He lost his ship and escaped with only a handful of his men. Such was his fame that backers lent him a new vessel, though a small one, and he enlisted a fresh crew. Eager for revenge on the Spaniards, he lurked among the cays on the north shores of Cuba, harrying the coastwise traffic.

The governor and captain general learned of his presence and sent a ship armed with guns and ninety men to destroy him. L'Ollonais stayed hidden, but made contact with the royal ship by means of boats rowed by buccaneers disguised as fishermen. The latter pretended to give the Spanish commander news of the notorious raider and pointed out a good anchorage for the night. Before dawn the war vessel was surrounded by these and other rowboats which closed in under the range of the cannon. L'Ollonais and his followers swarmed aboard, scoring an easy victory. All the surviving Spaniards were put to death, except one who was forwarded to Havana with the following braggart note to the captain general:

"I shall never give quarter to a Spaniard. I cherish the firm hope to execute on your own person what I did to those you sent with your vessel, the which was what you intended to do with me and my companions."

Yet l'Ollonais never struck at the Cuban capital. He transferred the skull and crossbones flag to his excellent prize and went elsewhere, to sack Maracaibo a few years later and finally to perish at the hands of Indians in Central America, who cut his living body to pieces slowly and are reputed to have eaten it.

Henry Morgan was a far more serious menace. An inspired leader of men, an able military strategist and political planner, he towered above the freebooting that brought him into prominence. He was to end with a knighthood and the governorship of Jamaica. Morgan had led the English buccaneers from Tortuga to Port Royal. In 1667 he was elected Admiral of the Brethren of the Coast in succession to Mansvelt. From then on, he sailed only under letters of marque issued to him by Sir Thomas Modyford, the third English governor of Jamaica, to whom he paid a share of the spoils.

Morgan had various rendezvous for his forces, one of which was the Isle of Pines. He was there in March, 1668, with twelve ships and 700 men, having conceived a plan to debark in the Gulf of Batabanó, march across country, and assault Havana on its unprotected land side. Esquemeling, the buccaneer annalist, who was present, reports that many of the corsairs had been prisoners in Havana, and these insisted that nothing of consequence could be done with fewer than 1,500 men. Cuban authorities assert, though the original documents in English do not mention it, that Morgan did put his troops ashore and start the march. Emilio Rig de Leuchsenring, the official historian of Havana, writes that the entire force landed at Batabanó and moved to enter Havana by way of the suburb of Jesús del Monte; but learning of preparations for defense, the chieftain abandoned the enterprise.

Be that as it may, Morgan took his ships around the west end of Cuba to Havana, passed the harbor mouth in slow defile, concluded that the Morro and other castles were too powerful to attack and returned to the south coast. He left the Havanese frenziedly digging trenches to resist him. Instead he marched inland to the city of Puerto Príncipe, now Camaguey, and gave it a thorough scourging.

As far back as 1655 a decision had been reached to protect Havana with a wall and moat. The work had actually been started, only to be given up because Spain had found other use for the funds promised. It was resumed in 1663, probably as a result of the l'Ollonais episode, and brought to completion in seventy-seven years. Even the beginnings

would have been valuable as breastworks, especially if linked
by trenches. I hold the theory that that was the deterrent
with Morgan as to the advance from Batabanó. Three years
later he performed a much greater exploit at Panama, but
he lacked the equipment in 1668, and the Puerto Príncipe
coup sufficed as a rehearsal.

The design of Havana's landward bulwark became plural.
There were to be walls in a polygon of nine bastions and
one half-bastion, united by escarpments and parapets, with
a covered way behind an exterior moat. One end was an-
chored on the La Punta Castle and the other on San Francisco de Paula. The ramparts enclosed at first a larger site
than had been built upon. Long before they were completed, the space was filled and overflowing.

816708

Chapter 6

HAVANA DROWSES BEHIND WALLS

THE WALLS typified, if they did not actually confirm
and mould, the isolation of the city under the mercantile
system of Spain. So it was with Cartagena de las Indias and
other walled places. Havana was now more orderly than it
had been, and the Church had somewhat more influence.
The Franciscans, Dominicans and Augustinians had large
convents. The Jesuits, who had come early, built in 1674 a
church on ground redeemed from a swamp near the Fuerza,

and this turned out to be the parent structure of the present cathedral. A nun named for the Magdalene had opened in 1635 a *beaterío*, or home for pious women, which expanded in a few years into the Santa Clara convent, still to be seen. The San Agustín, Cristo, and Angel churches were erected.

It had grown to be the custom of the bishops of Cuba, whose see was Santiago, to do as the governors had once done and spend most of their time in Havana. The machinery of the ecclesiastical hierarchy moved even more slowly than that of the state, and it would be many a year before two dioceses and an archbishopric were created. Rome frowned upon evasions. Several prelates were censured for being so little in Santiago, but the good men had their reasons, and these were not confined to the increased population of the capital. The Havana clergy often had to be disciplined for their loose behavior.

We read of a bishop complaining that some priests attended public balls and masquerades, thus exposing themselves to the temptations of dubious intrigues. Others found their clergy engaged in smuggling. A certain lay cynic remarked that the houses of prostitution were crowded most thickly about the monasteries and churches, as if seeking the proximity of a sure clientele. In spite of the constant ringing of church bells and the frequent religious processions in the streets—the favored route was along the Calle Amargura, a name meaning "bitterness"—the public was more addicted to debauchery than religion. From the middle of the seventeenth century, owners of Negro and mulatto slave women were known to send them out to solicit as prostitutes. The danger of getting killed in a gambling dive had lessened, but the number of such dives had increased.

The Inquisition had been introduced in 1634 and functioned spasmodically for a century. Heresy was its chief concern, with an admixture of vengeance on true believers who were personally distasteful to the inquisitors. Even the Holy Office needed popular support if its work were to be successful, and Havana was hardly the city to give that. So while an occasional auto-da-fé took place, there were few prominent victims. One old writer commented in the 1680's that "nobody, not even a Negro, has been burned for almost six months."

More serious was the growth of officialdom with all the evils that accompanied it in other Spanish colonies. Cuba had escaped the worst of this at the start because of its poverty and the shifting nature of its settlements, which tended to feed expansion in Mexico. The majority of immigrants were Spanish adventurers who could not yet be tagged as colonists, and they were an unruly lot. It would have been hard to make the men who had resisted the privateers feel inferior. The governors for the most part had been fighting captains of no social pretensions, some of them veterans of earlier New World efforts.

But as the island became productive, and especially as Havana flourished, grandees and generals regarded the chief-executive post as a plum. Lesser jobs, also, took on a seductive lure. Many thousands of those to be governed were now native born, and the shocking distinction between peninsulars and colonials common to Spanish America was sharply drawn. By the beginning of the seventeenth century in Cuba a colonial, no matter how well educated, could not be appointed to the meanest office, or obtain a military commission, or enter the priesthood, except as a rare favor granted by the highest authority in Spain. The few who were promoted paid hard cash for it and were forced to practice a degrading sycophancy. As a result the Creole developed intense local consciousness and rancor against the Spaniard. The latter retaliated with a grotesque scorn, expressed in the oft-repeated statement that a common sailor or ditchdigger from Europe was a superior being to an American-born landowner.

Havana drowsing behind its walls was less indignant about such things than the rest of the country. Its merchants were closer to the sources of power, and as individuals they prospered by it. They objected, however, to the tobacco monopoly set up by the Crown early in the eighteenth century, for tobacco was a strictly indigenous product which they had been handling free of duty. When the planters took up arms and seized Jesús del Monte just outside the city, Havana sided with them, but not for long. The three tobacco revolts, in 1717, 1721, and 1723, petered out and the monopoly nominally was absolute. A typical solution had been found. The weed thereafter was smuggled abroad from Havana in enormous quantities.

At the same period an activity got under way which was most pleasing to the city. The authorities in Spain decided to set up a yard near La Fuerza for the use of tropical hardwoods in the building of ships. The work was begun in 1724 and proved successful beyond all hopes. It was soon necessary to move the yard to the unoccupied, protected waterfront at the far end of the harbor, within the walls. It operated until almost the end of the eighteenth century, 114 ships being built there, including 51 ships of the line. This made the Havana yard the chief source—Humboldt called it the "great nursery"—of warcraft in the Spanish dominions. It was a royal enterprise, of course, but it created work for thousands and nice profits for local outfitters.

Spain and England were at war seven times in the eighteenth century, and the first four of these conflicts come within the scope of the present chapter. The first—the War of the Spanish Succession, which started in 1702—was of vast importance to the Caribbean region. It sprang from the fact that Charles II of Spain, called the Bewitched, died in

1700 without issue and was found to have willed the throne
to his Bourbon nephew Philip, a grandson of Louis XIV of
France. A Hapsburg archduke had a strong claim to the
succession, and England in alliance with Portugal and most
of the northern European nations backed him for fear of
the virtual merging of Spanish and French interests which
Philip represented. It was a grand-scale war lasting until
1713, but England eventually withdrew and the Bourbon
prince was confirmed as Philip V of Spain.

Exactly what had been anticipated took place. Spain and
France became friends. They supported each other for the
greater part of the century, until the outbreak of the French
Revolution. Havana was affected by this. It was passing
strange to its citizens to see French warships use the harbor
as a base, and to be invited to serve under French privateers
who had been given Spanish letters of marque. An expedition composed of French and Cubans sailed from Havana
in 1706, attacked Charleston, South Carolina, and brought
back plunder.

But the most interesting development of that war was the
recognition of French claims in Louisiana, a colony with
which Havana was thereafter to have close relations. The
brothers Le Moyne, known as the Sieur d'Iberville and the
Sieur de Bienville, had come from Canada in 1699 and
started the occupation of the Gulf Coast from Mobile Bay
to the Mississippi. At first Spain had resented the loss of
land which she had always claimed, though ineffectively
since the time of Hernando de Soto. With Bourbon Philip
on the throne in Madrid it was a different story.

Iberville, the elder brother, had left it to the youngster
Bienville to solidify the colony and later to found New
Orleans, and had gone on to wider activities as a French
naval commander. He had already fought the English successfully in Hudson Bay. Soon he was ordered to the Car-

ibbean to carry out an elaborate program, including the conquest of Jamaica. Iberville descended in March, 1706, on the small but important sugar island of Nevis, seized and devastated it, and carried off 3,187 Negro slaves. He disposed of his booty in Martinique, then went to Havana to organize a strong expedition. Fate stepped between this brilliant captain and the victories he might well have won.

While his flagship lay in the harbor, Iberville died on board of yellow fever in July, 1706. His body was hurried ashore the same day and buried in a church described as the cathedral. The edifice probably was the *parroquial mayor* dedicated to San Cristobal, restored after it had been gutted by the privateers in 1555, and doomed to be demolished when the palace of the captains general was built.

Havana saw little of Spain's next war with England. In April, 1727, during the third war, an English squadron blockaded the port. Its commander had failed to take into account the local shipbuilding referred to above. The defenders had a constant flow of craft from the stocks to launch against the enemy. At the end of a month the British had suffered heavy losses and were forced to withdraw, their admiral so mortified that he is reputed to have "died of grief and shame."

With the outbreak of the so-called War of Jenkins' Ear in 1739, Havana prepared for an attack by Admiral Edward Vernon. The latter struck instead at Porto Bello on the Isthmus, which he captured, and at Cartagena where he was disastrously repulsed. He suffered a lesser reverse in a move against Santiago de Cuba, and that was the end of Vernon afloat. The struggle merged into the War of the Austrian Succession. A few years passed. Then in October, 1747, a duel which most of the historians have missed took place in full sight of the Morro and Punta fortresses. Six Spanish and six English warcraft fought one another for six hours to a draw. They separated with losses set in round figures at one thousand men on each side, though one hundred is probably closer to the truth.

Quietly enough, the University of Havana was founded by monks of the Predicant Order on January 5, 1728. It was housed at first in the convent of San Juan de Letrán, and moved in 1742 to a convent yielded by the Dominicans which occupied the whole block between San Ignacio and Mercaderes, Obispo and O'Reilly streets. Public celebrations of this event were held. The subjects allowed to be taught were theology, jurisprudence, medicine, mathematics, philosophy, grammar, rhetoric, foreign languages, and canons of economic law. But this was a great advance over the curriculum set for the universities of Lima and Mexico in 1551, when the only studies permitted were theology, medicine, law, and ancient tongues.

There was no particular elation when the last stone of the walls was laid in 1740, for the moat and the covered way were incomplete. They would not be finished for another fifty-seven years. It would appear from ancient records that the enclosed city consisted of 179 blocks, fifty-six streets, three plazas, two general markets, one fishmarket, five private wharves, one general wharf, fourteen churches and convents, six military barracks, two hospitals, and one jail.

Chapter 7
CAPTURED BY THE ENGLISH

BACK IN 1665, in the days of the buccaneers, and only ten years after the English had seized Jamaica, a Major Smith of the British Army passed by way of Havana as a prisoner. He wrote a letter, which has survived and in which he said: "They [the Spaniards of Cuba] are so sensible of their weakness, and jealous of their riches in these parts that it is very difficult for any ingenious man, once taken by them, to get his liberty, fearing he might give such intelligence as would be the cause of their ruin. Witness their blindfolding of all strangers, when they pass their cities and castles, for they much dread an old prophecy among them, that within a short time the English will as freely walk the streets of Havana as the Spanish now do."

The value of the Key of the New World was, of course, fully realized in London. But Morro Castle continued to be forbidding until ships and weapons improved. After the defeat of Vernon at Cartagena, the English appear to have started to think seriously about Havana as the place where they might seek vengeance. In 1752 Admiral Sir Charles Knowles, who had fought with distinction under Vernon, was appointed governor of Jamaica and served for four years. According to Cuban authorities, Knowles visited Havana toward the end of his term, and instead of being treated with the suspicion described by Major Smith ninety years earlier, he was entertained by the captain general and shown everything. Knowles is said to have prepared a confidential report, as well as a plan of attack, for the English admiralty.

The Seven Years' War, in which England and France strove for colonial supremacy in the Americas and India, began in 1756. Spain did not take the side of France until the close of 1761, when her hand was forced by the treaties of the Family Compact under which the Bourbon monarchies obligated themselves to come to each other's aid. It proved a calamitous business for Spain. England immediately dispatched a powerful expedition to the Caribbean under Admiral Sir George Pocock, with General the Earl of Albemarle in command of the land forces. Its objective was Havana.

About forty warcraft of all classes assembled at Barbados. The troops under Albemarle were increased there to 11,000, and over one hundred transports provided. Jamaica had been asked to raise some 3,000 soldiers and the North American colonies 4,000. The middle of May the first Jamaica contingent of ships and men, led by Sir James Douglas, met Pocock off Cap St. Nicholas, Hispaniola, and the Admiral proceeded down the little-used Old Bahama Channel north of Cuba. He now had nineteen ships of the line.

The forces available at Havana to resist the attack are open to question. It is generally admitted that the population of the city at that time was around 30,000. Yet English estimates set the number of Spanish regular soldiers at over 4,500, the sailors on the ships in port at 9,000 and the militia at between 13,000 and 15,000 men, a total of at least 27,000, or almost as many fighters as there were inhabitants. The Spaniards said they had under 4,000 regulars and sailors combined, and arms for perhaps 3,000 militia. There were twelve ships of the line and three frigates on station. The condition of the Morro and Punta Castles was good, and the recently completed walls were fairly well manned. But the captain general, Juan de Prado, had worked out no general plan of defense.

Pocock and Albemarle had decided to strike from the eastern, or Morro, side of the harbor, which no enemy had done before. They had been correctly informed, possibly by the Knowles report, that failure to fortify the Cabaña ridge which lay parallel with the harbor, behind the Morro, almost nullified the value of the castle against such an advance. On the morning of June 6th the fleet was fifteen miles from Havana. Pocock sailed ahead with most of his warcraft, demonstrated in front of the harbor, and then made a feint of landing marines near the mouth of the Almendares River, as if that were to be his base of operations. Prado, tricked, hurried a strong force to the scene and the English marines were withdrawn. Albemarle, meanwhile, had put his whole army ashore, practically unopposed, at the mouth of the Cojima River, about six miles east of the city.

Havana perceived that it was in great peril. The church bells were rung and the people rushed panic-stricken about the streets. Prado created a council of war. There happened to be available a former viceroy of Peru and a field marshal who had been governor of Cartagena, both on their way back to Spain; as well as the chief admiral in American waters. This array of talent adopted three measures. The entrance to the harbor was blocked by the sinking of two large ships, all persons unable to bear arms were ordered evacuated, and the torch was put to the houses outside the walls. Needless to say, the evacuation could not be made complete at such short notice, especially since old people, women, and children had to be sent afoot beyond the burned suburbs. This destruction was necessary to prevent the English from using the houses as cover for an approach to the walls.

On June 11th, Albemarle assailed the Cabaña ridge—where a small redoubt had been thrown up in a hurry—and carried it easily. A battery of cannon was erected there, bringing both the Morro and the city under direct fire. Though Havana was heroically to endure a long siege, its doom had been sounded when the Cabaña was occupied.

The English soon had command of the countryside as well as the sea. They tightened the investment from day to day, began the bombardment of the Morro by Albemarle's batteries on the 20th, and on July 1st assaulted the castle from land and sea with their full force. Pocock brought three of his biggest ships as close as possible to the northeast side of the Morro, with orders to dismount its guns and smash its bulwarks. But the castle was held by a gallant and able commander, Luís de Velasco, a naval officer. At the end of six hours he had suffered terrible losses, while using his guns so well against the English that one of their ships was badly damaged and all had to be withdrawn. The respite was brief. The attacks were continued with growing intensity throughout the month.

Havana lost most of its fresh water supply when the *zanja*, or ditch, from the Almendares River was cut, an act which resulted in the flooding of large areas of the surrounding country. The roads, of course, had been closed and food could not come in from the plantations. As for the wonderful great walls, they proved to be badly constructed at many points, and although not carried they probably could have been. The policy of Pocock and Albemarle was merely to besiege and harry the city from the land side until the Morro had been taken. Few projectiles fell within the walls during that month of July. Four additional batteries, besides mortars, had been placed on the Cabaña; their bombs and grenades were poured steadily into the castle.

But the aggressors were not having a good time of it from any point of view. In addition to their military losses, yellow fever was causing untold havoc among them, with malaria and dysentery raging too. Albemarle obtained reinforcements from Jamaica more than once; they were needed sorely. He watched anxiously for the 4,000 troops that the North American colonies were supposed to send. Only 1,400 arrived, Colonel Israel Putnam leading a Connecticut regiment, and they did not land until July 28th.

On the 30th, a mine which sappers had skillfully laid under the south wall of the Morro was exploded. A breach was opened and the English went in with the bayonet. The Morro fell for the first and only time in its history. Albemarle had reserved the honor of heading the storming party for his two brothers, Major General W. Keppel and Commodore Augustus Keppel. His admiration of the brave defender Velasco, who had been mortally wounded in action, took the typical eighteenth-century form of graceful compliments and a suspension of hostilities on the day of the funeral.

Further resistance on the part of the city was hopeless, and Captain General Prado knew it. There had been rumors of the approach of a French squadron, however, so he held out for a while. The English now submitted Havana to a cataclysmic bombing. On August 11th, 6,000 projectiles burst amidst its narrow streets. Capitulation followed, and on the 13th the English marched in. The booty collected—they called it prize money—amounted to 1,882,116 Spanish dollars, worth about £736,180. Pocock and Albemarle each took £123,00, in round figures. The high officers under them received between £1,500 and £2,000, while common soldiers and seamen got an average of £4. Marked discontent was noted among the last-named.

Cuba was proclaimed to be annexed outright to the English Crown, though only the territory in the immediate vicinity of Havana had been occupied. Lenient terms were conceded to both the armed forces and the noncombatants. No seizing of private property occurred, at least not officially. The garrisons left in convoyed transports with the honors of war, the highest officials being given one of the captured frigates in recognition of their rank. Ordinary citizens had four years in which to decide whether to return to Spain or become British subjects. No change was made in the civil administration of affairs. The Catholic faith was guaranteed protection.

Friction inevitably occurred, most of it centering about the Church and the knotty personality of the bishop, Pedro Morel. He was furious when told that the bells of all the religious establishments would be taken as plunder, but arranged a compromise under which he paid 10,000 pesos and saved the bells. He properly objected to appointments in his diocese being subject to the approval of Albemarle, who was acting as governor. But the thing he found most scandalous was the demand enforced by Albemarle that one of Havana's churches be turned over to the English for the holding of Anglican services. Following a lively row, San Francisco was so converted, and since part of the premises was used as a cavalry barracks Bishop Morel declared that it had been permanently desecrated. Albemarle ended by deporting him to Florida.

The citizens complained about the quartering of troops and the many grievances of occupation. An armed uprising was planned, which led to executions of leaders. A small naval force that went to Trinidad de Cuba to take over was repulsed, and the town added an English red ensign as a trophy to its coat of arms.

Yet every Cuban authority agrees that the whole painful episode was a blessing to Havana. The Spanish system of a closed economy was overturned and bonds of all kinds were loosened. The English did not give free trade to Havana, because England herself did not practice it at that time; but having announced that the island was a colony, they allowed Havana to export and import goods under the English flag with few restrictions. The commercial markets thus opened were far more extensive than those afforded by Spain, and the taxes were lower. Intercourse with the Thirteen Colonies in North America was particularly lively. A number of merchants from New York, Philadelphia, and other Atlantic seaboard cities opened trading houses in Havana.

During the first ten months 900 merchant vessels docked at Havana, probably exceeding the total of the preceding five years. Many of them were slavers, but no one had as yet challenged the rightness of that traffic, and labor was needed. Eager purchasers awaited the blacks. The prices of sugar and tobacco boomed. Money circulated freely, and the mercantile class had little difficulty in reconciling itself to foreign rule.

If the English had remained, nationalist sentiment undoubtedly would have seethed dangerously against them outside of mercantile circles. But the Treaty of Paris signed in 1763 contained one of the most astonishing deals in the history of the Caribbean. England returned fertile Cuba to Spain and took low, sandy Florida instead. The sugar interests of Jamaica and the rest of the British West Indies had brought this about. They feared the competition in the London market which would have resulted from the full development of Cuban cane fields. As seen through the eyes of the military strategists, Florida was a poor exchange.

On July 6th, Albemarle evacuated Havana, leading his troops down the narrow Calle Obispo to the waterfront, while the Spaniards under General Alexander O'Reilly marched up the parallel street to the west, then called Sumidero, but which has since borne O'Reilly's name.

With the English gone, the people offered moral resistance so effectively to the old system of commercial strangulation that it had to be modified. Furthermore, the stimulated city almost immediately began to expand in a large way beyond the walls. For these reasons the English occupation is held to have been beneficial.

Chapter 8

HAVANA AND LOUISIANA

THE NEW CAPTAIN GENERAL of Cuba was the Count de Ricla, a prominent Spanish noble who had been given greater powers and a larger salary than had been attached to the office before. He may be said to have inaugurated the final line of rulers from abroad, most of whom were despots. Ricla himself was by no means one of the worst. General Alexander O'Reilly, who had come with him, was an Irish "wild goose," a graduate of Spain's Hibernia Regiment, whose military talent had carried him to the

top. He limped permanently from a wound suffered in the
War of the Austrian Succession. His present commission
was as inspector general of the forces in Mexico and the
Caribbean colonies.

Ricla and O'Reilly were charged with the task of insuring
Havana's future, the governor by improving the administration, the general by building new defensive works that
would really protect the city. Both did their jobs well,
though Ricla merely began measures which his abler successor Antonio Buccarelli carried out. O'Reilly was more
spectacular. He and the engineers under him designed and
began the castles of La Cabaña, Atarés, and Príncipe.
These fortifications were plainly indicated by the topog-
raphy of Havana's environs, the need of them proved by
the way the English had used the hills in question. Atarés
was completed in 1767, the great Cabaña fortress in 1774,
and Príncipe in 1779.

Meanwhile, O'Reilly had played a special role, the one
which has caused him to be significantly remembered in
the Americas. To salve the wounds of Spain in the Seven
Years' War, France had voluntarily ceded to her the city
of New Orleans and all that part of Louisiana territory
which lay west of the Mississippi, the part that had not
been lost to England. The transfer was intensely resented
by the French colonists, who resisted Don Antonio de
Ulloa, the first governor sent by Spain, and finished by ex-
pelling him. Ulloa, a distinguished scientist and explorer,
arrived in Havana with his suite and submitted a full report, for Louisiana had been made a province subsidiary
to Cuba. The news was forwarded to Spain, and time
flowed by while lackadaisical officials decided what should
be done.

At last, word came from Madrid. General O'Reilly was
to proceed to New Orleans with some 2,000 troops, take

over the government, punish the guilty and re-establish order. He moved promptly, with complete efficiency yet moderation according to the standards of the period. His flotilla of twenty-four vessels in July, 1769, overawed the French dissidents. Nicolas Chauvin de Lafrénière, the dynamic leader, was arrested along with eleven others. Six were sentenced to be executed, including Lafrénière, six to imprisonment and deportation. No action was taken against the many citizens who had supported the revolt. Compared with acts of repression elsewhere under the Spanish flag, the penalty exacted was mild indeed.

A French pioneer soldier and settler was made lieutenant governor. A *cabildo*, or municipal corporation after the Spanish pattern, was substituted for the administrative council, but all the members of the new body were French Creoles. A militia officered by leading citizens was established, and as soon as O'Reilly felt that it was functioning smoothly he sent most of his soldiers back to Havana. These policies won acclaim for the Irishman. He is said to have acquired Lafrénière's cook and to have shown no resentment when the slave threatened to poison him in vengeance. Such feelings were natural, he remarked, and sold the Negro to someone else.

One of his chief objects was to make the trade of Louisiana profitable to Spain. With this in view, he drove out large numbers of English smugglers who had been taking advantage of the unsettled state of affairs. He prevented the ships of all foreign nations from entering Louisiana ports, and he allowed heavy commerce only with Havana and Spain. However, he was not in full sympathy with the principle of a closed economy, and he persuaded the Council of the Indies in Seville that Louisiana should be permitted to buy and sell certain commodities without paying the usual heavy duties.

Also, O'Reilly made a notable exception in favor of a merchant named Oliver Pollock. This man, of Irish ancestry, had been a ship broker in Philadelphia for over twenty years at the time the English captured Havana. He moved down as soon as Albemarle declared the port open and did extremely well as a trader. The new administration under Ricla had of course ordered English merchants to leave, but Pollock made friends with O'Reilly, who got permission for him to go to New Orleans while that city was only nominally under the Spanish flag. It was the sort of favor that one Irishman might well do for another without any scheming for the future.

Apparently Pollock and O'Reilly corresponded, and we may assume that the former learned in advance about the latter's mission to Louisiana. A few weeks before O'Reilly came, Pollock had left for Baltimore where he loaded a large vessel, the *Royal Charlotte*, with flour and sailed back to New Orleans. The expeditionary force had landed during his absence, and the addition of 2,000 soldiers to a population of 3,000 had caused a serious shortage of food in the city.

Pollock immediately offered his cargo of flour at any price O'Reilly chose to set, averring that the humanitarian aspect was more important to him than profits. The governor allowed him a small margin of gain. In reporting this transaction to the Crown, O'Reilly recommended that Pollock be rewarded with a permit to trade freely at New Orleans in perpetuity, and it was granted. We shall find that this was by no means the end of Pollock's connection with Havana, Spanish governors, and the fortunes of the Thirteen Colonies.

Alexander O'Reilly was too big a man for a secondary colonial post. He had brought with him Don Luís de Unzaga, the colonel of the Havana Regiment, already commissioned as governor of Louisiana, installed him in December, but continued to supervise affairs until March, 1770. He then returned to Havana, to go on with his work of perfecting the defenses of the city.

An event which startled the Catholic world took place in 1767. This was the expulsion of the Jesuit Order from the Spanish dominions. The aggressive brotherhood founded by Ignatius de Loyola had had many disputes with state authorities and even with the Vatican. Portugal had driven it out in 1759 and France in 1762, but it was not thought that a country so devout as Spain would move against the strongest of all missionary propagandists of the Faith. The young king, Charles III, was supposed to admire the Jesuits. Yet his ministers persuaded him that they must be eliminated. Sealed orders were sent to governors throughout the Americas, not to be opened until a simultaneous given date. It is generally believed that the secret had leaked out, for the Order, or Society of Jesus, took the blow calmly. It had made arrangements for many of its fathers to "go underground" and escape expulsion.

All churches and other property were seized. The lands, nonconsecrated buildings and liquid treasure, worth millions of dollars, passed into the hands of the government. The churches were assigned by the bishop to priests of more subservient orders. It was at this time that the structure on the square off the Calle Ignacio became a favored place of worship under other than Jesuit auspices, though not as yet the cathedral.

On October 15, 1768, occurred perhaps the most catastrophic hurricane ever to strike Havana. In Spanish American countries these disasters are named after the Saint's Day on which they happen, and so the one in question is the Santa Teresa hurricane. Coming unusually late in the season, it took the people the more by surprise. A saying

current through the West Indies has been rendered in an
English jingle as follows:

> June, too soon.
> July, stand by.
> August, don't trust.
> September, remember.
> October, all over.

But the weather prophets were put to shame that October. The terrible wind of the circular tempest, moving
at a velocity which it was beyond the science of the period
to compute, smote the city with such force that whole
blocks of houses were torn apart and trees leveled as if
with a scythe. The sea was whipped into mountainous
waves that drove through the harbor mouth, and as they
ebbed carried with them the ships that had been lying at
anchor. The interior of the province over a radius of many
miles was turned into a snarl of wreckage.

Ironically enough, a hurricane has its useful aspects. It is
accompanied by torrential rains which soak the ground to
a great depth, and it gives the trees which stand up to it
a pruning they would not otherwise have had. Vegetation
consequently makes a quick recovery and is more lush than
before. The effect upon a city is to weed out the poorer
structures and thus stimulate improvement in the rebuilding. After the Santa Teresa storm an emergency use of
royal-palm bark for roofing was checked. Tiles, or the
alternative of flat Moorish masonry roofs, became obliga-
tory. The first official system of lighting the streets at night
was also adopted.

About this time the first practical division of Havana for
administrative purposes went into effect. The Count de
Ricla had set up four quarters. The plan was modified in

1770 by Buccarelli to two quarters—La Punta and Campeche—each to consist of four *barrios*, or districts. La Punta had the Dragones, Angel, Estrella and Monserrate *barrios*; Campeche the San Francisco, Santa Teresa, Paula and San Isidro. The derivation of only some of these names are clear, such as La Punta from the castle and others from churches. Campeche is a puzzle, for there seems no reason to have called a quarter in Havana after a small settlement on the Yucatan coast. Logwood, from which a dye is made, is campeche wood in Spanish, however, and as it is common throughout the West Indies at sea level it may have served to name the quarter. Santa Teresa may have been inspired by the recent hurricane, on the theory that the saint had guarded that district from total destruction.

Another municipal development was an assault upon the walls from within. The initial plan had provided for but two gates, one adjoining La Punta and the other at about the middle of the enceinte. The traffic of the growing city had found itself intolerably restricted. The merchants had demanded new gates, and by the year 1773 there were seven of them. It began to be earnestly suspected that the walls would crumble under cannon-fire in another siege, and that in times of peace they took up land that should have been used for homes and were a nuisance to business. Yet the government solemnly went ahead with the digging of the moat.

To all the defensive works, and particularly to the building of La Cabaña Castle, which cost 14 million dollars, the viceroyalty of Mexico contributed lavishly in treasure. The fall of Havana to the English had been a threat to Mexico which it was felt must never be allowed to occur again.

Chapter 9

THE AMERICAN REVOLUTION IMPINGES

In 1776 the breaking out of the American Revolution raised new problems for Spain in the West Indies. She dreaded the challenge to the monarchial idea, but even more was she anxious to see England weakened. Havana and its subsidiary New Orleans became centers of intrigue. The first and most active agent of the North Americans was that same Oliver Pollock whom O'Reilly had favored, and who was now a flourishing New Orleans merchant. Pollock induced Governor Unzaga of Louisiana to furnish privately 9,000 pounds of gunpowder from the royal stores. More help could not be obtained from this official, who was about to be transferred.

When the colorful, gifted young Bernardo de Gálvez arrived to succeed Unzaga in January, 1777, the latter told him that if Spain was going to side with Great Britain, "Oliver Pollock should not remain in the country twenty-four hours," but that if it were to be the other way about, the Irishman was the best foreign merchant for him to confide in. Gálvez at once became very friendly with Pollock, making him secret gifts of arms and medicines, and backing his credit. Yet Pollock was turned back when he tried to go to Havana at this time to extend his work for the Thirteen Colonies.

In 1778 France signed the Treaty of Amity and Commerce with the Americans and declared war on England. It was clear that Spain would join before long. This occurred in 1779. Gálvez seized the English forts on the lower Mississippi, then was ordered to take the leading part in the reconquest of Florida. The campaign was enlarged to include designs against the Bahamas and Jamaica, and Havana became general headquarters. A military man with a reputation, Don Juan Manuel de Cagigal, was appointed captain general of Cuba and arrived with a strong army. The building of new ships of war in the Havana yards was rushed.

After capturing Mobile on his way, Gálvez came to Havana to plan an assault on Pensacola, which was a well fortified place that received help from Jamaica. Among the officers assigned to him by Cagigal was a young Venezuelan named Francisco Miranda, the future precursor of Simón Bolívar in the great struggle for Spanish American liberty. Miranda took an active part in the reduction of Pensacola, which occurred in 1781. He was promoted from captain to colonel and placed in charge of clean-up operations in the Bahamas. Cagigal thought well of him and gave him an important post in the concentration of naval and military forces at Cap Français in the French colony of Saint Domingue, which were intended to join Admiral de Grasse in the conquest of Jamaica.

The crushing defeat that Admiral George Brydges Rodney administered to de Grasse at the Battle of the Saintes in April, 1782, put an end to that dream. Rodney gave England her only victories in the war and saved her Caribbean possessions for her. But when in August, 1782, he appeared off Morro Castle with twenty-six ships of the line, hoping to make an easy conquest of Havana, he found the city in complete readiness. Like Drake and Morgan, he contented himself with a demonstration and withdrew. He lacked the equipment to do as Pocock and Albemarle had done twenty years earlier.

Before peace was signed in 1783, Cagigal sent Francisco Miranda on a diplomatic mission to Jamaica, chiefly to arrange for an exchange of prisoners, partly to make an espionage agent's report on the island's defenses. Miranda returned to Cuba by way of Batabanó on the south coast, and was promptly accused by civil officials of having smuggled in contraband for his own benefit. It seems likely that Spanish jealousy of the advancement given a colonial-born officer lay behind the charge. Although Cagigal vigorously defended him, he was relieved of his duties and formally indicted. Miranda evaded the issue by fleeing to the United States, where he was welcomed by Washington, Jefferson and Hamilton. Thereafter he served republican causes, including that of the French Revolution, and tirelessly promoted the ideal of independence for all the Americas. His case was an example of Spain's folly in dealing with talented and ambitious young Creoles.

Oliver Pollock came back into the Havana picture, tragically for him, after peace was declared. A great sum was owed to him by the Continental Congress and certain state governments which he had aided with supplies. Requests for reimbursement were pigeon-holed. But, at his own request, he was given the appointment as first American consul at Havana. He was not violating the customs of the times when he loaded two ships with goods and planned to function as a merchant as well as a consul. The government in Cuba, however, professed to be indignant and delayed his landing by all possible means.

Spain, the ally of the United States in the recent war, presently went back into her shell of a closed economy and ordered all American citizens doing business in Cuba to pack up and leave. Pollock himself was arrested in May, 1784, thrown into prison and his merchandise seized because the State of Virginia had failed to meet a debt to certain traders of Nantes, France, the payment of which he had guaranteed with his signature during the revolution. Before long, all his personal belongings, including his carriage and his slaves, were confiscated.

Pollock was then released, but soon jailed again because of a document he had signed as one of the sureties for money that the Continental Congress had borrowed from Cuba and had not repaid. Luckily his friend Bernardo de Gálvez was transferred from Louisiana to the governorship of Cuba in 1785. Scandalized at finding Pollock in a cell, Gálvez gave his personal bond to obtain the release of the Irish-American, so that the latter could go to the United States and collect the sums due. It took until 1790 to negotiate a settlement. Pollock never returned to Havana, where he had been persecuted. The neglect and ingratitude shown him by his own country ran the maltreatment by the officials in Cuba a close second.

Charles III of Spain was a comparatively liberal monarch, but he was not capable of understanding the most intelligent of his ministers, the Count de Aranda. This statesman prepared a memorial in 1783, in which he prophesied that the United States would soon be formidable in New World politics, that it would wish to extend its territories and that it would grasp first for Florida. The King's colonial dominion, he said, was too large, too distant and too malcontent to be successfully defended if attacked by a strong power. Also, there might be revolutions against Spain, similar to the one against England. Aranda proposed that the colonies should be divided into three self-governing kingdoms, exclusive of Cuba and Puerto Rico which were

islands and could be safely retained. This was too much
for a king, even a liberal one, to swallow. The report was
filed away.

In 1788 Charles III died, to be succeeded by his dull
and reactionary son, Charles IV. A year later the Parisian
mob stormed the Bastille, and an upheaval greater than
Aranda himself would have dared to predict spread to the
Caribbean region. Following an abortive revolt of persons
of mixed blood in Saint Domingue, the black slaves there
rose in 1791 to demand their liberty under the French
Revolution. Toussaint l'Ouverture emerged as their leader.
The planters gradually were overwhelmed by numbers,
and many of them took refuge in Cuba.

Aranda's memorial was dug out of the filing cabinet and
reconsidered. It was even more distasteful to Charles IV
than it had been to his father. Rule the colonies more
strictly, root out sedition, punish the friends of republican
France: that was the decision. In Havana it simply had
the effect of opening the door to some charming but un-
distinguished members of the French *ancien régime*. Elsewhere it stimulated premature conspiracies, and as the
upshot of events in Hispaniola the Spanish half of the
island had to be turned over to France. Tens of thousands
of Negro slaves, some of whom had had French masters
and some Spanish, were successfully transferred from Hispaniola to Cuba.

Despite the nature of the regime in Madrid, Cuba had
the luck to be governed through most of the 1790's by a
good and enlightened man. This was Luís de las Casas, a
protégé of General Alexander O'Reilly, who had recommended him for the post. He had been a soldier, and at
forty-five had risen to the highest rank, but was as yet without experience as a civilian administrator. Not much was
expected of him by the people of Havana.

Las Casas raised the standard of education. He subscribed from his own purse to the founding of a number of public schools. Grotesque as it may seem, Cuban girl children had been forbidden until his time to learn to read. He sponsored a biweekly newspaper called *El Papel Periódico*, amusing and liberal in sentiment compared with its only predecessor, which had been a semi-official gazette. He encouraged a native theater which produced light comedies of Cuban life, while more serious works were brought by touring companies from New Orleans. Operettas featuring the dance became extremely popular.

The Patriotic Society, to use the popular contraction of its long and flowery name, was undoubtedly one of the best works of Las Casas. He established it in collaboration with the ablest and most well-to-do residents, Cubans as well as Spaniards. Its object broadly was to develop the island's resources, including the arts and sciences as well as farming and industry. Though benighted governors of the future showed it small consideration, it stayed alive and served a good purpose whenever the atmosphere was favorable. Through its agency and otherwise, the famous reformer Francisco de Arango, who was born in Havana, was able to get mercantile concessions from the Crown from time to time. He even had the port opened for a short period to foreign trade.

A census under Las Casas—probably the first one that had been honestly taken—showed the population of Havana and its suburbs to be 44,337. In the whole of the island there were some 273,000 inhabitants.

The palace of the captains general, begun in 1776 on the site of the original parish church, was sufficiently ready in 1790 for Las Casas to move into it shortly after he had assumed office. It then filled the southern frontage of the Plaza de Armas, and part of it was assigned for use as a

prison. Finishing touches were more than forty years distant.

As his term drew to a close, Las Casas participated in an
event which still causes idle dispute. The bones of Christopher Columbus and his son Diego were supposedly transferred from Spain to the cathedral of Santo Domingo in
1542. When the Spaniards gave up the colony to France,
they insisted on taking the remains of the Discoverer with
them. A leaden casket, which is said to have borne no inscription, was dug up and removed to Havana on the war
vessel *San Lorenzo*. The bishop, captain general and other
officials received it ceremoniously, and it was placed in a
wall of the chancel of the new cathedral, formerly the
Jesuit church. This occurred in January, 1796. But in 1877
excavations in the cathedral crypt of Santo Domingo revealed a sealed coffin marked with the name and distinc-
tions of the elder Columbus. As the grave of Don Diego
was not found, in spite of a careful search, I see little
reason to doubt that it was his bones that the Spaniards
took with them by mistake.

Chapter 10

LIFE IN THE EARLY 19TH CENTURY

HAVANESE LIFE, as the eighteenth century merged
into the nineteenth and for a full generation afterward, had
a unique flavor. The people felt the mental impact of

Homeric events, notably the revolutions against Spain that followed the American and French revolutions. But they themselves were not called upon to suffer. Havana was the only large Spanish colonial town that was physically untouched, and amidst the crashing of thrones and the birth of constitutions it became a clearinghouse. The upper class enjoyed great luxury, for Cuba was growing sugar cane, tobacco, and coffee profitably, while the rest of the empire ran blood from 1810 to 1824. The lower elements had some share in the general prosperity; they developed a singularly wild bohemian spirit, and the forms of lawlessness that Havana had always loved—gambling, wenching, brawling —were never more salient.

There were those who grumbled that the liberal regime of Las Casas, rather than the news from abroad, should be blamed for turning the city's head. He was even reproached for the fact that in 1800 the craze for dancing had become almost a mania. Havana then had in excess of fifty dance halls open to the public, but only a single respectable one "by subscription" for families. Be that as it may, the documentation on what did go on is much fuller than for any preceding period. Famous travelers as well as natives have left memoirs.

In December, 1800, Baron Alexander von Humboldt, historian, geographer and naturalist, one of the most eminent men of his epoch, arrived for a visit of three months. As a result he wrote his *Political Essay on the Island of Cuba*, as part of the chronicle of his scientific journeys through the Americas. The views he expressed were considered of such importance that he was hailed as "the second discoverer of Cuba." Humboldt found much to delight him from the start. He wrote that the entrance of the port of Havana was "one of the gayest, most picturesque and enchanting vistas" that could be seen in the New World north of the Equator. "The European gets so alluring a series of impressions here," he adds, "that he is likely to forget the danger with which the climate menaces him. . . . He contemplates those great fortresses built on ridges, the mountains to the east of the city, that shell of the sea [the inner harbor] surrounded by villages and ranches, the city itself whose narrow and dirty streets are half hidden by a forest of the masts and sails of vessels."

Later he remarked with disgust that Havana needed to be properly policed: "I walked through mud to the knees, and the many carriages or *volantes*, which are the typical carriages of this city, and the drays laden with boxes of sugar, their drivers rudely jostling the passerby, made walking in the streets both vexatious and humiliating."

Humboldt and his companion, the scientist Bonpland, were the house guests of the rich Cuesta family. They were entertained by practically every person of social importance, including the Marquis de Someruelos, the new captain general, and were taken on trips throughout the island. But Humboldt was not the man to be deluded by flattering snobbism. He formed his own opinions, denouncing Negro slavery as the curse of the country and predicting a sound economic future when it should be abolished. Also, as a sworn bachelor who was fond of women, he amused himself freely. One of his biographers says that years afterward a Cuban went about claiming that he was a son of Humboldt. The Baron shrugged the youth aside with the remark that he was the fifth false pretender to that paternity.

Humboldt took keen interest in the fortifications. He declared that with war raging in Europe, the coast of Mexico must be counted "a military dependence of Havana." He left in a schooner for South America, but his vessel which sailed from Batabanó was forced to put in at the port of Trinidad de Cuba and he spent two days there. His second and last visit to Havana occurred in 1804, when he stopped over for about a week on his way from Veracruz to the United States.

Café life, bullfighting, cockfighting, and other sports, which had been moderately popular before, took a sudden spurt at this time, competing with the dance. True, there was only one important café, La Dominica, on the Calle Mercaderes between the captain general's palace and the cathedral, but many little ones were opened in all parts of the city. The fame of La Dominica increased from decade to decade throughout the better part of the century. The bullfight, a Spanish rather than a Cuban sport, remained on an amateurish level because the local animals usually showed up poorly in the ring. Contrariwise, the cockfight had always been one of the island's pursuits, and now excellent strains of gamecocks were bred.

Decent women, of course, had no part in all these diversions. Apart from church and the theater, they could appear in public only for formal drives in the afternoon, called *paseos*. Their favorite rendezvous was the Alameda outside the walls, not known as yet as the Prado, which ran down to the sea. Observers, both native and foreign, consistently made mild fun of the custom, though admitting its elegance. The women sat with heads and shoulders bare in their low, long-shafted carriages or *volantes*, plying their fans, bowing to the occupants of other vehicles, and accepting the homage of gentlemen on horseback with whom they were acquainted.

A critic wrote in 1805: "The *paseo* has been reduced to making a million turns in the *volantes* from mid-afternoon to sunset around the fountain and to the Alameda. At least we must be thankful that we can contemplate the ladies with their arms of alabaster, laying bashfulness aside and facing the elements." But he went on to condemn their

excessive use of make-up. The large number of smart
women to be seen did not come only from the wealthy
merchant class. Planters and cattle ranchers had taken to
building town mansions where their families spent as much
time as possible.

The same critic looked into the ways of lesser folk and
thought many of them fantastic. He was struck by the
popularity of *velorios*, the Hispanic equivalent of wakes.
"They have become outright fiestas," he comments, "to the
extent that the writer found himself in front of a house
where a corpse was laid out and a friend of the deceased
said to him: 'Come in and amuse yourself at the *velorio*,
where there is enough to eat and drink for all who may
come.'"

Havana had long been noted for an overplus of slaves,
especially females, for each member of a household had to
have his or her private attendant in addition to general
servitors. This was in part a social vanity, in part a catering
to licentiousness among the men. The same roof sheltered
legitimate family life and the most wanton sex relations
between masters and slaves. The offspring of mixed blood
usually were freed. The newspapers of the period were
filled with advertisements of young Negresses for sale, described in a set formula as "good washerwomen, healthy,
and without blemishes," who could be had at from 250 to
300 pesos. A sturdy female field hand, however, was worth
about 400 pesos.

It might be supposed that under these conditions there
would have been little scope for public prostitution except
of the cheapest sort. Such was not the case. The calling
flourished, though less wildly than later in the century after
the emancipation of the slaves. There was a demand on
the part of the well-to-do for European harlots. Captain
General Las Casas had promoted immigration from the

Canary Islands in 1792, with the effect of augmenting the number of white prostitutes though it had been far from his intention to do so. A special prison, the Casa de Recogidas, had had to be established for female offenders, most of whom were of the demimonde.

In 1808 Napoleon invaded Spain, forced the abdication of Charles IV and his heir Ferdinand, and placed Joseph Bonaparte upon the throne. This sensational coup plunged the colonies in the New World into political confusion, and paved the way for independence. Cuba was perhaps the least affected. The officials, supported by rich Creoles, swore allegiance to the young prince as Ferdinand VII despite his father's action. Frenchmen were declared to be enemies. Most of the Saint Domingue refugees were expelled, with disastrous results to the economy of Santiago province, where they had increased the production of coffee tenfold. Because of these steps Cuba as a whole had long to bear the disgrace of being called by Spain the "Ever-Faithful Isle."

The revolutions in Venezuela and Mexico broke out almost simultaneously in 1810. Their meaning grew slowly on Havana, centering about the supreme name of Simón Bolívar, a subject with which I shall deal in the next chapter. Hidalgo and Morelos, the Mexican patriot priests, were almost incomprehensible to Cubans. Lesser matters appeared to be of more immediacy, anyhow.

Cuba had been created an archbishopric in 1804, with bishops in both Santiago and the capital. The following year, Bishop Espada of Havana ended the burial of bodies inside the churches and founded the first ecclesiastical public cemetery. The story goes that until 1805 all graves were in the churches, but that can hardly have been the case in view of the growing population and the comparatively small number of churches. That all funerals of any distinction were so conducted is indisputable, and the sanctified crypts had become charnel houses from which diseases spread. To prevent ostentation, the bishop forbade special monuments and even the private ownership of the lots in his cemetery, but as he was induced to make exceptions for officials and corporations his "equality in death" was soon an empty phrase.

A census which appears to have been fairly reliable, taken in 1810, showed that the population had swelled to 96,114, an impressive figure for the period in the New World, and only 259 less than that of the city of New York.

In 1812 the gambling spirit was turned to the profit of the state by the establishment of the first lottery. The institution has been so widely patronized ever since that you find it hard to believe that Havana could ever have been without it. The original price for a whole ticket was sixty cents and the top prize $500. As the earnings from the start were around 40 per cent, both the stake and the rewards boomed progressively.

Also in 1812 there began a period of political liberalism, short but marvelous, which threw the minds of thinking men into a turmoil as optimistic as that with which the lottery had imbued the devotees of luck. A nationalist junta in Spain had held out against Napoleon, and with the aid of an English army under Wellington was making it impossible for Joseph Bonaparte to cling to the throne. A parliament which met at Cadiz adopted a constitution under which the colonies were freed of many disabilities. This was regarded as so much talk by the provinces already in revolt. But Cuba hailed the news with joy, especially as certain autonomizing laws were put into effect.

Two years later Ferdinand VII was restored. He was a despot and a viciously stupid one, who lost no time in abrogating the Cadiz constitution. However, the old state of affairs could not be brought back at once, and until 1823 there was a seesaw of oppression and tolerance. Newspapers bearing provocative names, such as *El Sabelo Todo—o el Robespierre Habañero* and *Los Rugidos de un León Africano*,* were published almost without interference at times, were savagely censored at others. Intellectuals flocked to La Dominica Café and uttered the sentiments of Voltaire and Rousseau.

Thousands of middle-class families, both upper and lower, ignored politics and passed a tranquil existence inside the walled city. Away from the waterfront and the commercial streets where the traffic had irritated Humboldt, all travelers agreed that the atmosphere of Havana was dreamy and quiet. *Cecilia Valdés*, by Cirilo Villaverde, which Cubans regard as *the* national novel, contains some admirable pictures of life in the Angel district at this epoch. The action of the book opens in the year 1812 with a mysterious visit paid by a gentleman of quality to a modest street and house which are described as follows:

"The narrow lane of San Juan de Dios is composed of only two blocks, closed at one end by the walls of the convent of Santa Catalina and at the other by the houses of the Calle de la Habana. The hospital of San Juan de Dios, which gives it its name, and through the high square windows of which comes perpetually the warm fume of the sick, fills the whole side of the second block. The other three have little one-story houses with red-tiled roofs and one or two stone steps at the door. Those that make the best appearance are in the first block, entering from the Calle de Compostela. They are all of the same size more or less, with a single window and door, the latter of cedarwood studded with large nailheads painted the color of

---

* *He Knows Everything—or the Havana Robespierre; The Roarings of an African Lion.*

brick. The street remains in its primitive and natural state, is stony and without sidewalks. . . .

"There was very little furniture in the parlor [of the house visited]. Against the right-hand wall stood a mahogany table upon which burned a wax candle in a bell-glass shade. And there were several massive cedarwood chairs with seats and backs of leather fastened with copper nails, this sort of thing being regarded as luxurious at the time, and much more so in the case of a woman of color such as the one who occupied that dwelling as a mistress and not as a servant."

Chapter 11

THE SUNS AND RAYS OF BOLIVAR

ON HIS FIRST VOYAGE to Europe, as a boy not yet sixteen, Simón Bolívar touched at Havana where his ship was in port for two days. Being a member of a Venezuelan family that had been ennobled, he carried letters of recommendation to the captain general and doubtless was received. But we have no knowledge of his impressions. The year was 1799. His career as liberator was well advanced before he even mentioned Cuba, along with Puerto Rico, as units in his vast program of Spanish American independence.

The next occasion when the Bolívar name figured in

Havana was marked by equivocal circumstances. Maria Antonia, a sister of Simón, had criticized some of his policies. This made her suspect to the revolutionary government in Caracas and she was expelled from the country, though not by Simón's orders. She came to Havana in 1816, where she found herself gravely embarrassed financially and is said to have had to work for her living. She then took the sad step of asking the Spanish Crown for a pension, which Ferdinand VII promptly granted and later doubled. The king signed a document in which he spoke of the persecution suffered by his loyal subject Maria Antonia Bolívar because of her constant opposition to revolutionary ideas. It was good propaganda from his point of view.

Nevertheless, the persecuted one returned to Caracas within five years, taking her first opportunity to do so. Simón merely reproved her in affectionate terms and gave her property back to her. She supported him thereafter.

Bolívar shortly after the start of his Peruvian campaign wrote a letter to his vice-president in Colombia which contained the phrase: "I am like the sun, sending out rays in all directions." This letter was made public and reached Cuba with extraordinary rapidity. There already existed several secret societies which hoped to bring about a revolution. The most important of these took the name of the Suns and Rays of Bolívar, derived moral force and a fresh appeal from the appearance of being linked directly with the Liberator, and became powerful. It planned an uprising, to be launched at a given hour in Havana and various interior points on August 16, 1823.

Early that year Francisco Dionisio Vives had arrived as captain general. He was a great fancier of gamecocks, which did not prevent him from improving the espionage system of his predecessor, while wooing those citizens whom he called *sensatos*—the prudent ones—detesters of change on the theory that it would endanger property rights. Agents of Vives wormed their way into the membership of the Suns and Rays. The arrest and ruthless punishment of the leaders broke up the conspiracy. Among those to escape with the light penalty of banishment was José Maria de Heredia, Cuba's first notable poet and possibly her best. Padre Félix Varela, the distinguished priest, philosopher, educator and statesman, who was representing Cuba at a constituent Cortes in Spain, had to flee the country. He took refuge in the United States and ended his days at St. Augustine, Florida.

The Spanish government now abolished all the privileges that had remained over from the liberal constitution of 1812. Cuba was placed under martial law. New taxes were imposed to pay the costs of heavily increased garrisons. These steps were mild compared with the reaction to Bolívar's triumph in Peru in December, 1824, which ended Spanish rule on the North and South American continents. The Liberator intimated that he had troops available for descents on Cuba and Puerto Rico, and that in certain circumstances he would send them. Madrid then issued the Royal Order of May 29, 1825, under which Cuba was administered, with modifications of small import, until she at last won her independence at the end of the century.

The captain general was advised that he was invested "with the whole extent of power which, by the royal ordinances, is granted to the governors of besieged towns. In consequence thereof, His Majesty most amply and unrestrictedly authorizes your Excellency to remove from the island such persons, holding offices from the government or not, whatever their occupation, rank, class, or situation in life may be, whose residence there you may believe prejudicial, or whose public or private conduct may appear suspicious to you, [etc., etc.]."

All elected law-making bodies were done away with. The *cabildos* or municipal councils were emasculated. The right to bear arms, except in the service of Spain, was denied. Political meetings of any description became illegal. One highly vexatious ordinance provided that no man might entertain a stranger overnight at his house without previous notice to a magistrate. The entire expenses of government, civil, military, and religious, were to be drawn from taxes and customs duties. Surplus revenue, if any, would be remitted to Spain.

Yet Cubans continued to plot, in the hope of intervention by Simón Bolívar. The latter, with few ships at his command, hesitated over the proposed Caribbean adventure. At times he felt that he could get quick results, at others that it was a forlorn hope. Then a scheme for a joint expedition by Gran Colombia and Mexico took shape, and this was the one that came closest to being carried out. Bolívar heard that Mexico might be willing to furnish 6,000 men and some ships. In 1826 a tentative agreement was signed by the two new republics. A logical policy emerged: Colombia would direct its main efforts against Puerto Rico, which had long been used by the Spaniards as a base that menaced the north coast of South America. Mexico would invade Cuba, with which its military fortunes had always been linked.

It turned out to be only a bright dream, of course, but one that had other phases before it was relinquished.

The question of the future status of the islands arose. If they were taken from Spain, would they be set up as republics? Or would Cuba be annexed by Mexico, Puerto Rico by Colombia? No decision was ever announced. But the mere debating of it was enough to stir the United States and Great Britain to diplomatic action. Both powers let it be known that they did not wish to see any change of sovereignty in the islands. What the United States really meant was that she regarded Cuba as territory she would eventually acquire, and she preferred that ideas of autonomy should not be fostered there. Britain meant that if she was to retain her own prestige in the Caribbean, the flag of discredited Spain was the safest flag to have flying in Havana. Neither Washington nor London cared about Puerto Rico, except that it was thought just as well to lump it with Cuba.

Bolívar was most anxious to be favorably regarded by the two Anglo-Saxon powers. He met the views of Henry Clay and George Canning halfway. Yet in 1827, when he went to Venezuela to heal dissensions there, he again took up the problem of the Antilles and agreed with General José Antonio Páez that the latter should lead his idle army of more than 10,000 men to Cuba and Puerto Rico, whether or not Mexico gave support. The Liberator is believed to have been worried by the large concentration of malcontents in Havana, fugitives from his regime who were joining in the oppression of Cuba and who might organize raids against him. The plan came to nothing, as did some lesser ones. With Bolívar's fall and exile, and his death in 1830, the island patriots abandoned hope of aid from the continent.

Havana became more cynical than it had ever been, more contemptuous of law now that it had been deprived of even the minimum rights of citizenship. Men who would have given their lives for their country scornfully risked the garrote as smugglers, robbers and assassins. Some, to be sure, were relieved at having been spared the choice of sides in an insurrection, because they sincerely dreaded the Negro problem.

One of Bolívar's pronouncements had been that if he came he would emancipate the slaves. But in no country where he had done this was the proportion of blacks to whites as large as it was in Cuba. The island was supposed to have some 800,000 inhabitants, though there were probably more. Admittedly a maximum of 45 per cent were of pure blood, and the number of light-colored free persons who had thrown in their lot with the ruling caste and were accepted as whites brought the total to only a little over 50 per cent. There may have been 100,000 free Negroes and mulattoes, and 300,000 slaves, the latter figure being much open to question since there was a head tax on slaves, and proprietors consistently reported fewer than they really owned. The situation was not comparable to that of French Saint Domingue, where the blacks and free colored had outnumbered the whites eight to one. Race animosity existed in Cuba nonetheless, and a civil war for control was feared, should there be a sudden emancipation.

Commercially, Havana had wrong but all too human reasons for hoping that slavery would not end in Cuba. Its prosperity turned on a large and growing traffic in African Negroes which Spain tolerated. None of the great powers had given up human bondage. But England in 1807 and the United States in 1808 had abolished the slave trade. After the Napoleonic Wars ended, these two countries had conceived it to be their duty to take naval action on the high seas and in the Caribbean to prevent the "black ivory" from being shipped to the New World. They soon had to contend with a revival of piracy, as well as illicit slaving, for freebooters hijacked the vessels from Africa and sold the seized freight. The environs of Havana became the chief clearing house. The best ultimate market was the southern part of the United States.

Now Spain had not joined in outlawing the trade. Up till 1820 she furiously protested Anglo-Saxon interference with the landing of captive Negroes in Cuba and Puerto

Rico. England finally bought off Ferdinand VII for £400,-
000, and that venal monarch proclaimed the traffic ended in
Spanish dominions north of the equator. He still laid claim
to colonies in South America, but was nearing defeat there.
The act applied, in effect, to Cuba and Puerto Rico. Part
of the bargain was the appointment of two commissioners,
one English and one Spanish, to be stationed in Havana
and supervise its enforcement. The thing was a farce on the
Spanish end. Slavers were given secret protection, and instead of paying taxes as of old, they shared the profits with
the authorities.

The township of Regla on the eastern shore of Havana
harbor grew to be a main headquarters of smugglars and
pirates. By 1830 thousands of dollars per week flowed from
their activities through the hands of dock-owners, merchants and purveyors of entertainment. The forehead of
Our Lady of Regla, the especial patron of seamen and
boatmen, is credited with perspiring miraculously, a faculty
that may well have been acquired at that period.

One of the captains general is said to have collected half
a million dollars for his benevolent attitude during a four-
year term toward Regla and other centers of contraband.
The semi-official Bank of San Fernando openly discounted
the notes of slave traders at 10 per cent. Insurance companies issued policies covering the voyage to Africa. The
English commissioner protested in vain.

Not much of this graft seeped down to Havana's poor,
but their own lawlessness was winked at—so long as they
did not talk politics.

Chapter 12

TACON, OR THE HEEL

FROM THE LONG LIST of Cuba's tyrannical governors, two or three are remembered because their personalities were strange and their regimes sensational. Probably the most notable of these was General Don Miguel Tacón. His family name means "heel," the heel of the foot, but fits him aptly if rendered in American slang. He had served in the wars against Bolívar, and according to rumor he had been mutilated in battle in the manner he would have least preferred. Therefore Tacón hated colonials, apart from his conviction that they were inferior beings politically.

He was appointed captain general in 1834 as a strong man who would put an end to crime. In view of the vast powers of his office under the royal ordinance of 1825, he had been given a ready-made dictatorship which he proceeded to wield in a highly personal way and with a brusqueness to which Havana was unaccustomed. This was not just what the Court had wanted. Ferdinand VII had died, unregretted, in 1833 and had been succeeded by his three-year-old daughter, Isabel II. The regency of the dowager queen, Maria Cristina, had promptly been challenged by the first Carlist movement which claimed the throne for the late Ferdinand's brother, an extreme reactionary. Civil war broke out. Maria Cristina needed the support of

77

liberals. Her mandate to Tacón was to reform Cuba, not to set up his own brand of justice in a private satrapy. She soon discovered how bizarre a choice she had made.

Even those who most deplored Tacón admitted that he stamped out the kind of wrongdoing that showed on the surface, cleaned up Havana physically, and instituted great public works. This has always been the stock program of a dictator who values credit at least as much as plunder, who wants to leave a name in history. One of his first moves was to take over from the municipality the right to name the under-commissaries of police. His men really disarmed the underworld, seized or silenced every disturber of the peace from footpads down to beggars. His sanitary squad forced citizens to observe a rigid code and extirpated the roving dogs half-mad with hunger which had grown to be a serious peril. Gambling houses were censored, those which harbored criminals being suppressed. For the first time, no doubt, the streets of Havana became perfectly safe for pedestrians by day or night.

Tacón's way of getting quick results, however, left much to be desired. He insisted upon a minimum number of arrests in each district each week, and he placed army officers in the courtrooms supposedly to protect the magistrates but actually to see that they found the accused guilty and imposed stiff sentences. At the slightest sign of weakening, he summoned his policemen and harangued them savagely. "The more unwarrantable the acts of his subalterns the more acceptable to him, since they, in his opinion, exhibited the energy of his authority," writes Gonzalo de Quesada. "They trembled in his presence, and they left it to persecute, to invent accusations, to imprison and spread terror." Bloodhounds were employed to track suspects.

Larger evils were handled differently. Tacón denounced the slave trade, piracy, and all that went with it. When approached by dealers he heaped public contumely upon them. But he appointed private agents to let them know that they must observe outward decorum while continuing to pay a heavy tariff for protection. It was no part of his plan to deny himself the juicier spoils of office. He is said to have piled up a greater fortune than any of his predecessors.

When he had what he wanted—a smoothly running machine and the appearance of virtue—Tacón started to build and to beautify the city. He it was who put the finishing touches to the palace of the captains general. He gave it a marble portico facing on the Plaza de Armas, removed the jail to a huge new structure near the Punta Castle, and devoted the whole of the old premises to governmental and ceremonial purposes. Tacón reconstructed the Alameda, or Prado, into a handsome tree-shaded avenue with driveways on both sides, and called it the Paseo de Isabel II after the child queen. He created a broad avenue running from what was then the outskirts of the city to the foot of Príncipe Castle, naming part of it for Charles III; it soon came to be known as the Paseo de Tacón. A splendid theater was erected and named the Tacón, but its true builder was a smuggler with whom I shall deal presently. He gloried in receiving homage for all these things.

The captain general also posed as a Harun al-Rashid, a beneficent caliph who was informed of everything and used original means for protecting the oppressed. Many stories along this line are told of him. He is said to have learned that a certain man had been falsely imprisoned for debt, to have had him released by paying the sum out of his own pocket, and then simply to have notified the real debtor who his present creditor was. The account was thereupon settled with record speed—and Tacón announced it to the populace.

The most celebrated anecdote concerns Miralda Estralez, a beautiful young orphan who kept a cigar store and was engaged to marry a worthy boatman named Pedro. Count Almonte, an aging roué, set out to seduce her. Since she would not listen to his offers of money and jewels, he kidnapped her and took her to his country estate. How she managed to preserve her virginity in such circumstances is not revealed, but the tale has it that she did. Pedro discovered her whereabouts and complained to Tacón, who sent soldiers to bring both Miralda and the count to him. A stern inquisition was held, and when he had satisfied himself that Almonte had indeed kidnapped Miralda the captain general ruled that the two must be married at once. He summoned a priest, watched the ceremony performed and then dismissed everyone without further explanations.

Pedro felt justifiably injured. Had he not acted in time to save his sweetheart from ravishment? Why should the villain get her, after all? But Tacón's constructive duplicity soon became clear. On its way home the Almonte party was waylaid by soldiers disguised as bravos, who killed the count. Miralda, married yet intact, inherited as his widow and was enabled to endow her second husband, Pedro, with a large fortune. No guarantee of truth accompanies this story, though it has appeared in numerous chronicles.

Two years after Tacón assumed office he got a chance to play the tyrant in a big way and made full use of it. The re-establishment of the constitution of 1812 had been forced upon Maria Cristina by her own party in Madrid, and Cuba was necessarily advised. The mail vessel made its first stop at Santiago, where the provincial governor, General Manuel Lorenzo, received his copy of the orders.

Lesser officials had been honored in the past for zeal in such matters, so Lorenzo at once issued a proclamation and commenced reforms. Tacón was furious. He bluntly announced that the royal decree of 1825 empowered him to do as he saw fit, and that for the island's good he refused to apply the constitution.

He sent a flotilla with troops against Lorenzo, drove him into exile and arrested hundreds of persons who had supported the provincial governor. Doubtless with his tongue in his cheek, he granted the single point that deputies to the Spanish Cortes could be elected. One of these was José Antonio Saco, of Santiago, Cuba's outstanding advocate of Negro emancipation. When the deputies and Lorenzo reached Madrid they were repudiated. The supposedly reform parliament passed the following resolution:

"The Cortes, using the power which is conceded to them by the Constitution, have decreed: Not being in a position to apply the Constitution which has been adopted for the Peninsula and adjacent territories to the transoceanic provinces of America and Asia, these shall be ruled and administered by special laws appropriate to their respective circumstances."

Tacón had won. His policy of ruling Cuba by stamping on the native whites and favoring the free colored element, as a means of widening the breach between Spaniards and Creoles, was fully approved in Spain. Shortly after he had defied the new constitution he was promoted in military rank. He is reported to have said, "I am here not to advance the interests of the people of Cuba, but to serve my master, the Crown." On another occasion he even admonished the sovereign, "You shall never hear the petitions of your American vassals contrary to my pleasure." Anything resembling a free press had been throttled by him, of course, and the schools had been censored. Yet José de la Luz y·

Caballero, one of Cuba's greatest educators and a political revolutionary at heart, began the significant phase of his work under Tacón.

An observer from the United States, R. B. Kimball, described Tacón as a man "in whom shortsightedness, narrow views and a jealous and weak mind were joined in an uncommon stubbornness of character." It is dubious whether Don Miguel's mind could be termed weak, and his shortsightedness was by choice; he was determined to get results while he reigned. José Martí, Cuba's noblest patriot, wrote a generation afterward: "Tacón governed the island like a lord of the manor, loosing dogs at the men and ships at the generals who obeyed the national law that he trod underfoot."

Oddly, one of Tacón's most devious transactions was with another Martí, or Marty, a contrabandist of that name, also known as the "King of the Isle of Pines." The slave trade had no monopoly of smuggling, and the ordinary commercial kind was seriously affecting the revenue from customs duties. Bribes were being paid to lesser officials, but not enough of this money reached Tacón. He ordered a campaign of repression, which failed utterly. Captain Francisco Martí, operating from the then almost uninhabited Isle of Pines, landed goods at will up and down the coast and sold them through the dealers of Regla within Havana harbor. Tacón offered rewards for evidence against the smugglers, and an attractively large sum for the person of Martí.

Choosing a cloudy night the outlaw, who was tall, dark, and agile, slipped between the two pacing sentries on guard at the front entrance of the palace and coolly mounted the marble stairway to the first floor. He nodded to another sentry, giving the impression that he was an accredited visitor, and entered the private office of the captain general. Tacón, writing at a desk there, did not take the intrusion in good part until assured that his caller could furnish full information on the methods and hiding-places of the contrabandists.

"Prove it," said Tacón drily, "and you'll have no difficulty about collecting your reward."

"I must first know that your Excellency will pardon me, no matter what my offences may have been, if I live up to my boast in the present matter."

"I pledge you my word of honor," the other said.

"All right—I am Captain Martí."

For once Tacón was taken aback. But the situation was of the kind that appealed to his acid humor. He had the smuggler chieftain locked up for the rest of the night, and in the morning turned him over to the coastguard squadron as a guide. Martí systematically revealed his past practices. He allowed boats and depots to be captured, but not his faithful followers who presumably had had advance warning from him. When brought back to Havana he had performed his end of the bargain. Tacón gave him the pardon and the reward. Martí, however, handed back the money. "I suggest that you keep that for charitable purposes," he said. "What I should prefer instead is a monopoly of fishing rights and the sale of fish in Havana. I am willing to build a public market at my own expense, which shall be an ornament to the city and which after a term of years shall revert to the government." There is no documentary proof that he also proposed a share of the profits for the captain general, but this is accepted as a matter of course. The deal went through.

This episode is a favorite in Havana lore, because it shows up Tacón as a heel from whom the initiative was seized by a clever Cuban rascal. We do not have to believe it in all its details. Something of the kind happened. The ex-smuggler established his fishmarket on the Calle Mercaderes near the cathedral and prospered fabulously. Then he turned his talents to the entertainment business. Under Tacón's protection he built the theater which he called after his patron. It stood outside the walls, at the upper end of the Paseo de Isabel II and facing what is now the Parque Central. One of the largest and best-equipped theaters in the world, it flourished for generations as the home of grand opera, drama, and public balls. "This will amuse the people and keep their minds off matters which do not concern them," Tacón remarked to a group of friends when its doors were opened.

He was recalled to Spain in 1838 after having served four years of a five-year term. Nothing justifies the supposition that he had fallen into disfavor. He probably had grown tired of living in fear of assassination, concluded that he had made enough out of Cuba, and felt sure that he would never be forgotten. When he left, jingles were sung in the streets. The following is a free translation of one of them:

> If you mixed up together
> Cataline and Tarquin
> With the sultans of Algiers,
> Adding Tiberius and Nero
> And the Holy Inquisition
> And Attila's mad fury;
> Then with iron and human blood
> You kneaded such a mess:
> You could make in miniature
> The great Tacón of Havana.

Chapter 13

THE FIRST INSURRECTIONS

REGIMES LIKE Tacón's serve to bring to a head the rebellion which they sought to avert. Successive captains general, particularly two of some note, Leopoldo O'Donnell and José de la Concha, had well-merited trouble on their hands. But Havana, as was always to be the case in Cuba's struggles for independence, did not prove to be the center of action. The merchant class clung to its policy of "business first," and the poorer citizens were laggard. The thinkers found it necessary to take their ideas elsewhere. It was to be a long time, in fact, before many Cubans either in the towns or the countryside could believe that it was possible to end Spain's misrule without help from abroad.

Havana in the 1840's was a self-indulgent place which enjoyed the material improvements made by Tacón, while frankly pleased to be rid of his burdensome presence. A good picture has been left by the Comtesse de Merlin, who was born Mercedes de Santa Cruz on the Calle Cuba in the capital about 1794. She was a precocious, adventurous girl who developed into a brilliant woman. Committed to the Santa Clara convent by her father, because he felt that she needed discipline, she escaped and fled to Spain where she joined her mother at the court of the pseudo-king, Joseph Bonaparte. Not long afterward she married a French

85

general with a title and became a social figure in Paris. She wrote and sang with distinction.

The Comtesse de Merlin revisited her native city in 1840, the result being a book of impressions which was first published in French in 1844. She spoke of the luxury of the life, partly due to the large number of slaves. Some families even lent one another their slaves on occasion for purposes of ostentation. Coming straight from France, she was as astonished as an alien-born might have been at the sun-smitten total calm of midday during the hours of siesta. "Follow me through the streets of Havana at one in the afternoon and you will find no life, no noise, no movement," she writes. "The dust of Herculaneum and Pompeii is not more fiery, nor the place more of a desert. But indoors love goes on, and little else."

The women of her world began to return to outdoors activity in the late afternoon: "At six all the *quitrins* wait at the doors of the houses. The women sally forth with bare heads and natural flowers in their hair, and the men with dress-coats, cravats, white waistcoats and pantaloons. One by one the *quitrins* go down the Paseo de Tacón, and here and there dash the *volantes* which well deserve that name."

The *quitrín* was a new development, perhaps the most graceful carriage ever invented. The ceremonial *volante*, not the vehicle seen on country roads, was often drawn by two horses with a postilion on one of them, their harness ornamented with silver and the traces drooping. The *quitrín* had a body like that of a victoria—balanced between two immensely large wheels that came higher than the hood when it was thrown back—and long shafts with a single horse well forward from the back of which a coachman in livery wearing a top hat directed the equipage. A *quitrín* full of ladies, every detail of their costumes visible, resembled nothing so much as a laden flower-basket bobbing on delicate springs.

All aspects of city life interested the Comtesse de Merlin. She found the custom of the *velorio* just as popular as it had been at the beginning of the century. Arriving too early for a wake, she overheard a conversation that was touched with macabre humor. Should the dead man wear pink or violet drawers? a feminine voice asked plaintively. Neither, came the austere reply, for he was to be in the robe of a Franciscan brother. Shortly afterward the *zacateca*, or undertaker, produced his masterpiece, and the ritual of mourning lightened by lavish refreshments began around the coffin.

"There is no populace in Havana; there are only proprietors and slaves," she writes, with something less than accuracy, though the spirit of her meaning is clear. "The first are divided into two classes: the land-owning gentry and the mercantile middle class. The last-mentioned is composed for the greater part of Catalans, who, arriving without patrimony in the island, end by making great fortunes. They begin to prosper by their industry and thrift and at last get possession of the finest hereditary estates, as a result of the high interest at which they lend their money."

She has a sentimental view of slavery and recounts many anecdotes to prove that the blacks enjoyed their condition. For instance, there was the slave who had worked on holidays until he had collected enough cash to ransom himself. He asked his kind master what price he set upon him. The answer was: "Nothing. You are free from today!" The Negro looked silently at his master for a moment, wept, and went off. A few hours later he returned, bringing with him a fine *bozal*, or newly imported African, whom he had bought with the sum intended for his own freedom, and said: "Your Honor had one slave before; now he has two." A likely story.

It is true, however, that the Spanish code covering human bondage was comparatively lenient. It gave the slave the right to have himself valued by a magistrate and to insist upon emancipation if he could pay for it. Lacking the price, the slave could compel his master to transfer him to any other person who was willing to meet the terms fixed. The uncertainty of black labor supply caused the government to begin the importation of Chinese coolies on eight-year contracts in 1847.

In the early 1840's, immediately after the Comtesse de Merlin had left, there were a number of small servile revolts which the authorities bloodily repressed. Free persons of color showed their sympathy with these movements, a fact which Tacón must have learned with disgust. The caste produced a martyr in the person of the mulatto poet Valdés, who wrote under the name of Plácido. He was the illegitimate son of the Spanish dancer Concepción Vázquez and a colored hairdresser. His mother deposited him at the Real Casa de Beneficencia, Havana, a charity founded by Bishop Valdés in the previous century, where unwanted children were received without questions asked, taught a trade and sent out into the world bearing the name of the founder. So this boy became Diego Gabriel de la Concepción Valdés. He carved tortoise-shell combs for a living. When he began to write at an early age he adopted the *nom de plume* of Plácido.

Some of his published verses boldly declared his love of liberty. He also circulated political opinions in manuscript. So it was not strange that he fell under suspicion and was arrested in 1844 when a new slave uprising was feared. His trial, however, was a burlesque of justice. He was hurriedly convicted and shot with nineteen others at Matanzas, at the age of thirty-five. On the way to the place of execution he chanted his last poem, which began: "Stay Thou, O Lord, the oppressor's victory!"

Captain General O'Donnell was then building the lighthouse at Morro Castle, as a monument to his administration. It became a torch and a symbol of the city in Cuban hearts, few structures being pictured more often, and it might well be counted a memorial of the death of Plácido.

Conspiracy along ambitious lines and with a remarkable leader now followed. General Narciso López was of Venezuelan birth, yet had risen to the highest rank in the Spanish army. His wife was a Cuban, and after living in the island for some years he grew to abhor the injustices practiced. He did not believe that Cuba could stand alone. The course that had been taken by Texas appealed to him. First a successful revolution to earn the respect of the world, and then an application to the United States to be admitted as a full-fledged state. He began to plot in 1847. Many rich landowners supported him at first. The movement was betrayed to the Spaniards the next year, and López fled to New York. Cirilo Villaverde, the novelist, also a fugitive, became his secretary.

López at once received offers of backing, chiefly from Southern slave-holding interests who felt that the acquisition of Cuba would strengthen their own policies in the Union. President Polk's government announced that it was willing to buy for cash. Madrid replied that sooner than transfer Cuba to any other power, Spaniards "would rather see it sunk in the ocean." That proved to be a tremendous advertisement for López, who enlisted several hundred North American adventurers. He offered the command first to Senator Jefferson Davis and then to Major Robert E. Lee. They declined, but were sympathetic.

The first López expedition sailed from New Orleans in 1850, flying the flag of the single star which was to be adopted when Cuba became a republic. After touching at Yucatán, a descent was made at Cárdenas. It turned out to be a fiasco because the idea had not been sufficiently promoted in the island and the people failed to rise. López took refuge at Key West. He was charged with filibustering, but the case was dropped.

Again he recruited a force, this time including 150 Americans with military experience, under Colonel William S. Crittenden of Kentucky and others under Colonel Robert Wheat of Virginia. Striking directly from New Orleans in August, 1851, a landing was made at Bahía Honda, fifty-five miles west of Havana. López committed the error of dividing his little army. He advanced toward the capital with some 300 men, leaving Crittenden to organize a rear. Though López won skirmishes and inflicted heavy casualties, he was finally beaten. He and Crittenden were captured with the majority of their troops. Wheat escaped.

The Spaniards treated the prisoners with ruthless brutality. Crittenden and some fifty North Americans were shot without a trial at Atarés Castle, López condemned to be garroted at La Punta. The general asked for an interview with Concha, the new governor, who had served under him in the Spanish army and whom he had promoted. The request was coldly denied, and López perished in the grip of the iron collar. His last words were, "My death will not change the destinies of Cuba."

As a matter of fact, his execution put the seal of permanence upon the national cause, especially as another martyr was bracketted along with López. Joaquín de Agüero had risen in Camaguey, had read a declaration of independence, and checked the Spanish troops sent against him, only to be overwhelmed later and put to death. The governor of

Santiago province gave a banquet in Bayamo to celebrate these events. Speeches gloating over the end of Narciso López had been made, when a young man burst into the hall and delivered a violent address. He condemned the affair as being in bad taste and, carried away by anger, let fall certain phrases which revealed his sympathy for the beaten revolution. He was Carlos Manuel de Céspedes, member of an influential Bayamo family, a planter, lawyer and poet.

They treated Céspedes as a mere hothead, confined him and two of his friends who had become implicated, and then freed them with a reprimand. It was a blunder from the standpoint of the authorities. For Céspedes was to prove a far more effective patriot leader than López had been.

Chapter 14

THE TEN YEARS' WAR

SEVENTEEN YEARS were to pass between the defense of General Narciso López uttered by Carlos Manuel de Céspedes and the latter's emergence on the plane of action. The revolutionary spirit marked time during those seventeen years. In any study of Cuban history it is important to place Céspedes accurately, so we shall look backward for a paragraph or two. He came to Havana at the age of sixteen to study at the Real Seminario de San Carlos, a college

which then had more prestige than the university and was
thought to suffice for the education of rich youths. The year
was 1835. Céspedes, being ambitious, passed on to the university in 1836 and graduated there as a bachelor of laws
early in 1838. He remained for still another twelve months
in the capital.

The period, except for a few weeks at the end, was that of
Tacón's government. No political ideas were being openly
discussed among intellectuals. The students, watched nar-
rowly by agents of the tyrant, did not even have a bohemia
where they could forgather. Céspedes had the entrée to
good society and could not have failed to enjoy himself. His
youth resembled that of Simón Bolívar, but we know nothing about the forming of his mind in Havana. He figured on
none of the lists of suspects furnished to Tacón.

On returning to Bayamo at twenty, Céspedes was a gay,
elegant man of the world, who fenced expertly, played chess
and wrote verses to pretty girls. He married one of his cous-
ins before he was of age, but less than a year afterward
surprised his family by leaving alone for Spain, to pursue
further studies at the University of Barcelona. He found the
old country torn by intrigues against the queen regent,
whose side he was inclined to take because she was supported by the Spanish liberals. More to the point was his
friendship with a unique personality, General Juan Prim,
destined to be briefly dictator of Spain, and whom he believed to be sympathetic to Cuba.

In 1844 Céspedes went on a grand tour of Europe. The
country whose institutions most impressed him was England, and Turkey the only one where he observed misgov-
ernment to be compared with that of Cuba under the
Spaniards. Apparently he was not inspired by his journeys to
strike for liberty, as Bolívar had been. He came back to his

easy life at Bayamo, to the rearing of children, and was not heard from significantly as a patriot until he defended the memory of Narciso López. That episode behind him, he again lapsed into a long silence.

The chroniclers tell that the cities, and notably Havana, experienced their most opulent days in the decade and a half that followed the López disturbances. Great new mansions were built by sugar planters and other rich men. The Aldama palace outside the Havana walls cost $400,000, a more important sum at that time than it would be now, and it took $30,000 to furnish the drawing room. But the income of the Aldama family was currently estimated at $3,000,000 per annum.

Many North American, English, and French visitors came to Cuba in the 1850's and some have left books about it. The writers included Richard Henry Dana, Jr., author of *Two Years Before the Mast*, and Julia Ward Howe the poetess. Local memoirs appeared, such as José Maria de la Torre's *Lo que Fuimos y lo que Somos*. Havana journalism improved, at least in the matter of presenting descriptive and human-interest material.

Dana's was the best of the travel books in English. It was published in 1859 under the title of *To Cuba and Back*, and it has lasting vitality as a picture of Havana. On landing from his ship, Dana skirted the Plaza de Armas and remarked in nearby streets "the dead walls of houses, with large windows grated like dungeons and large gates showing glimpses of interior courtyards. Horses and carriages and gentlemen and ladies and slaves all seem to use the same entrance. The windows come to the ground, and being flush with the street and mostly without glass nothing but the grating prevents a passenger from walking into the rooms." That might be said of parts of old Havana today. But Dana records vanished nuances: "We drove through the Puerta de Monserrate, a heavy gateway of the prevailing yellow or tawny color . . ." the reference being to the walls.

His hotel, Le Grand's on the Prado, had no bathroom, so he visited a public bathhouse: "We must go through a billiard room where the Creoles are playing at the tables and the cockroaches playing under them, and through a drinking room and a bowling alley; but the baths are built in the open yard, protected by blinds, well ventilated and well supplied."

Dana enjoyed still more the seabaths a little to the west of La Punta and the Prado. He describes them as "boxes, each about twelve feet square and six or eight feet deep, cut directly into the rock which here forms the sea-line, with steps of rock, and each box having a couple of portholes through which the waves wash in and out." Open to the public without charge, these baths and others farther up at the Torre de San Lázaro existed until quite recently.

Among the eminent travelers was William R. King, elected to the vice-presidency of the United States with Franklin Pierce. He took the oath of office at Matanzas in 1853, an ailing man who died within a few months. The next year tense diplomatic relations over Cuba occurred between Spain and the Union because of the astonishing "Ostend Manifesto" drawn up at the Belgian seaside resort by the American ministers to England, France, and Spain. ·These gentlemen recommended that $120,000,000 should be offered for Cuba, and if rejected "by human and divine law we would be justified in wresting the island from Spain." Nothing came of the manifesto, though one of the signers was James Buchanan, who was to be the next President. Gradually the bad blood engendered cooled down.

The War of Secession in the United States made Havana a center of illicit commerce between 1861 and 1865. At the same time it put an end to the slave trade with Dixie, and this large market having been lost, with the rest of the region. Few Spanish ships attempted to run the Federal blockade, but goods collected in Havana were supplied to the adventurers who sailed from Nassau in the Bahamas. The city was an important haven for refugees as the war drew to an end. Confederates were much more popular in Cuba than Federals. Judah P. Benjamin, who had been Confederate secretary of state, arrived after a strange odyssey in a buggy through Florida and put up at the Hotel Cubano, where he found General John C. Breckinridge, ex-secretary of war, General E. Kirby-Smith and other notables. A fairly large number of Southern "irreconcilables" were given residence permits by the colonial government.

It chanced that the middle of this period of conflict in North America was the time selected for the destruction of the now quite useless walls of Havana. The change was authorized by an order from the Crown in 1863; the first section demolished was between Obispo and O'Reilly, the space being preserved as a square under the name of the Plazuela de Albear.

Peace had barely been restored in the United States when Spanish despotism was challenged from two quarters. In Spain itself a revolt against Isabel II failed in 1867, but was successful the following year under General Prim, and the queen was driven into exile. This was the juncture chosen by Cuban nationalists at the eastern end of the island to strike the first great blow for independence. Carlos Manuel de Céspedes had never ceased to feel reproved by the example of López. He had gradually built up about him a circle of patriots who knew what they must do when the opportunity offered. At first Francisco Vicente Aguilera was even more active than Céspedes and was regarded by many as the leader.

Spain had appointed in 1866 a sort of fact-finding commission to which delegates from Cuba and Puerto Rico had
been invited. The Cubans had stated as their minimum de-
mands local self-government under a constitutional system,
freedom of the press, and unrestricted industrial liberty, and
had been bluntly told that these could not be granted. Yet
new taxes were at once imposed and the proclamation so
worded as to make it seem that the colonial delegates had
approved them. Thousands of Cubans offered passive resistance to the tax collectors. It was an issue that bit deep,
especially in view of the growing political disturbances in
Spain.

Apparently with some foreknowledge of what Prim was
about to do and hoping for justice from that leader, Céspedes seized the initiative and called a meeting of thirty-six
important sympathizers at his sugar plantation, La Dema-
jagua, Santiago province, on October 9, 1868. Armed revolution was decided upon. This became a fact the next day
with the so-called Cry of Yara, when an action was fought
at a village near the scene of the death by burning of
Hatuey, the Arawak cacique, at the hands of the first Spanish conquerors. The slaves were declared emancipated. Céspedes, then forty-nine years old, was elected provisional
president of the Republic of Cuba. An uprising followed in
the adjoining province of Camaguey, its outstanding chieftain being the gifted Ignacio Agramonte.

This was no flash in the pan. It was the beginning of the
terrific struggle known as the Ten Years' War. The possibly
good intentions of Prim in Spain were nullified by his assassination. The Spanish government adopted savage measures, and after its troops had been decimated it sent out
General Arsenio Martínez Campos, its ablest commander.
On the Cuban side military talent of a high order developed. A volunteer from Santo Domingo who enlisted with

the grade of sergeant was before long a general; his name was Máximo Gómez. Another foreigner, General Thomas Jordan, a former Confederate officer from Virginia, was for a short time in 1869 and 1870 supreme commander of the Cuban revolutionary troops. Antonio Maceo, the great mulatto chieftain, and Calixto García won their spurs in campaigns cruel beyond belief, a hell of reprisals. The Spaniards devastated the countryside and shot every male found away from his home. The *insurrectos* retorted with guerrilla tactics, including machete charges both afoot and on horseback such as European troops had never conceived and which outdid the use of the lance.

But serious fighting never came west of the center of the island and Havana was little affected by it. A revolutionary junta existed under cover in the capital; it had plans for coups in all the western provinces, and for a while Céspedes counted upon its activities. The harshness of the Spanish regime at the seat of power, the difficulty of land communications with the east, the selfish fears of the mercantile class: all these factors kept Havana inactive. That is not to say that there were no individuals who made sacrifices. Bloody clashes between citizens and Spaniards in uniform occurred at the Villanueva Theater and the Louvre Café. Hundreds slipped away into the bush to join the patriot army. Miguel de Aldama gave most of his huge fortune to the revolution. After it was learned that he had gone to New York as an agent for the Céspedes government, Spanish soldiers wrecked and looted his magnificent new palace referred to previously; they left it a shell, which later was converted into a tobacco factory.

In 1869 a lad of sixteen, born of poor parents in Havana, came under suspicion for having published a poem which seemed vaguely seditious. Then it was discovered that he had been one of the signers of a letter rebuking a school companion for having enlisted in a Spanish regiment. For these offenses the lad was condemned to six years at hard labor and put to work in a stone quarry with iron shackles on his legs. In a few months friends got the sentence commuted to exile, at first in the Isle of Pines, and soon it was interpreted to allow him to go to Spain. He was José Julián Martí, the greatest of Cuban leaders, who would one day organize the successful War of Independence.

I do not have the space to give details of the long-drawn-out conflict in eastern Cuba. At the end of five years in office, Céspedes was forced out and a number of short-term provisional presidents succeeded him. A few months afterward he was trapped in a mountain retreat by Spanish troops and killed. At about this time the *Virginius* incident almost involved the United States in war with Spain. A blockade-runner commanded by Joseph Fry, a former Confederate officer, and carrying munitions and recruits for the Cuban forces, was seized near Jamaica by the Spaniards and taken to Santiago de Cuba. The crew and passengers of the *Virginius* were all charged with filibustering. Their trial was a farce. Captain Fry and fifty-two others were shot, and further executions were prevented only by the intervention of Sir Lambton Lorraine, commander of a British sloop-of-war, who threatened to bombard the city if the slaughter was not stopped. Many of the victims were North Americans and intense rage spread throughout the Union. Yet Washington contented itself with protests.

For Havana the supreme incident was not that of the *Virginius*, but the judicial murder of eight medical students brought about by the *voluntarios*, a loathed body of Cuban soldiery in the service of Spain. Gonzalo Castañon, a colonel of *voluntarios*, edited a paper in which he grossly slurred the people of the island and at last printed an article insulting to Cuban women. For this he was challenged to a duel and killed. His body was placed in a vault of the old cemetery founded by Bishop Espada. Months passed, and then forty-three students were arrested on the complaint of a soldier and accused of having desecrated the tomb.

At the court martial of the boys, the youngest of whom was only sixteen, Captain Federico Capdevila, a Spanish officer, conducted their defense and obtained an acquittal. But the *voluntarios* insisted upon a mistrial, and at a new court martial all the accused were found guilty. Eight received the death sentence and the others imprisonment for life. A second Spanish captain, Nicolás Estévanez, protested courageously that the affair was an outrage, but neither he nor Capdevila could prevail against the *voluntarios*. The eight students were shot against the wall of the commissary building that faced La Punta Castle, the date being November 27, 1871.

The corpses were thrown into a ditch in unconsecrated ground. Unfortunately for Spanish honor, a son of the editor Castañon made a journey from Spain to examine his father's tomb. He declared that it had never been tampered with. In due course the Spanish Cortes conducted an inquiry, voted that all the students had been innocent and released the survivors from jail. It was too late. Nothing that the oppressors had ever done was remembered with more bitterness than the slaying of the eight young martyrs.

Also in 1871, the poet Juan Clemente Zenea, captured while attempting to take the wife of Carlos Manuel de Céspedes to safety, was executed by a firing squad in the Cabaña fortress.

General Máximo Gómez and other leaders in the field met with reverses during the last five years of the war. Agramonte was killed in action. On the level of statesmanship the guiding hand of Céspedes was grievously missed. But resistance died slowly. Martínez Campos finally talked the

Cubans into a peace by making many rosy promises. The Pact of Zanjón was signed in 1878, after the Spaniards had lost 208,000 men and the Cubans about 50,000. It was but a truce. The abolition of slavery, however, can be ascribed to that part of the heroic drama that had already been staged. The Spaniards proclaimed the reform in 1880 and carried it into full effect in 1886.

Chapter 15
GAIETY AND CORRUPTION

THE TEN YEARS' WAR confirmed a mood of cynicism which had been present in the life of Havana in the 1850's, and after the defeat of the national forces it grew more marked. Superficial prosperity returned to the capital and with it a feverish gaiety. But everyone knew that the east was ravaged, starving—a thing to put out of mind since it could not be remedied. The Spanish military flaunted their power, a subconscious fear of "the next time" in their hearts, while the civilian officials hurried to enrich themselves, scornfully refusing to make even a pretense at good government. The native-born either played along with the conquerors and got a mean share of the profits, or kept up the appearance of neutrality. Both peoples laughed with their lips only. A few Cubans continued to plot in desperate secrecy.

Demolition of the walls was still proceeding in 1878, though nearing the finish. A journalist of the times used the figure of speech that the old thoroughfares had long since overleapt the barrier and prolonged themselves: Obispo as San Rafael, O'Reilly as San Miguel, San Juan de Dios as Neptuno, and so forth. The lines were not traced with precision, yet it is a fact that San Rafael, for instance, was almost a continuation of Obispo and had become the great shopping street of the new quarter as its parent had been of the old. To be sure, there were differences. San Rafael was much the wider, and its atmosphere was that of Paris and New York rather than of a Spanish colonial city. Dress, jewelry, and perfume shops crowded one another; on the block between Consulado and Industria stood Mme. Ragusa's Museum, which exhibited curiosities similar to those of the famous Barnum's in New York. The broad crosstown avenue named Galiano was the most outlying center of smart shopping.

The theater was extremely popular. A constant flow of traveling companies from Spain, France, and the United States gave operas, dramas, and variety shows. The great Adelina Patti was among those who came in opera. The Tacón, which seated 3,000, remained the finest house from every point of view; additional decoration had given it a wealth of cut glass, gilt, and colored velvet. Its nearest competitor after 1877 was the Payret, completed early that year on the upper Prado by a Catalan impresario named Joaquín Payret, and which seated 2,500. Other prominent theaters were the Albisu, noted for its one-act comedies of Spanish life; the Jané, which combined circus attractions with the drama; and the Villanueva, a repertory house.

The chief sport was of course the cockfight, mains being held every Sunday in several pits on the outskirts and drawing impassioned audiences. The bullfight was increasingly regarded as a Spanish spectacle, which Cuban patriots avoided not because they thought it cruel but because it was Spanish. The chief bull ring was at Regla across the bay, a wooden amphitheater that seated 10,000 spectators. Another large ring stood in town at the foot of the Calle Belascoain near the ocean front, the site being part of the present Parque Maceo. The Basque game of *jai-alai*, or *pelota*, was played by amateurs; it was by no means the rage that it has become in modern Havana. Baseball, introduced from the United States in the late 1880's, was slowly winning favor. The newspapers referred to it as "a hygienic sport."

Dancing had lost none of its appeal, and as the population at the end of the Ten Years' War was estimated at being 300,000 within a six-mile radius of the center of Havana, the number of dance halls had greatly increased. It achieved its most spectacular form at the masked balls held in the winter months at the theaters, particularly the Tacón, during the Christmas season and Carnival. Richard Henry Dana had written in 1859 of such an affair: "The music is loud and violent, from a very large band, with kettledrums and bassdrums and trumpets; and because these do not make noise and uproar enough, pistols are discharged at the turns in the tunes." Later, however: "The drums and trumpets were hushed, and all had fallen as if by the magic touch of the approaching dawn into a trance of sound, a rondo of constantly returning delicious melody, as nearly irresistible to the charmed sense as sound can be conceived to be—just bordering on the fusing state between sense and spirit. It is a contradanza of Cuba. The great bells beat five over the city, and instantly the music ceases. The watchmen cry the hour, and the bells of the hospitals and convents sound their matins, though it is yet dark."

Dana's dance had taken place in a hall next to his hotel on the Prado. In the 1870's, though the character of the music was similar it was usually rendered by military bands, and if the scene was the Tacón the utmost splendor prevailed. The parquet of the theater was built up temporarily to the level of the stage and the entire space below the great chandelier made into a dancing floor. Five tiers of boxes and balconies swept in a horseshoe converging on the stage. All was thrown open to the public, except for certain privately owned boxes reserved for parties that supposedly intended merely to be observers. As the overwhelming majority of those present were in costume and masked, the opportunities for intrigue were boundless.

Respectable women did not attend, or at least denied that they would dream of doing so. There were many stories of clandestine forays in impenetrable disguises. The regular clientele of the masked balls were men about town, the more pretentious cocottes, and women of mixed blood who had no social position to lose. The rule of the mulatto beauty was a phenomenon of the times. No matter what the shade of her complexion, she was called "Mulata," the word being used in friendly greeting. Not all of those who took part in night life could properly be listed as cocottes. Many were the recognized mistresses of white men, and some were professional dancers or singers. In his study of Havana in the mid-nineteenth century, De la Barras writes of the caste as follows:

"They are in general indolent and care only for creating a situation for themselves in which they may enjoy luxury and amusements. They are apt to be spendthrift and vain. Their liking for the dance amounts to a frenzy; they prefer it to all other diversions. At balls they are possessed by an ardent vehemence that manifests itself by voluptuous and exciting movements, not deliberately intended to be shameless as with public women, but as the result of a natural, restless impulse and the fire of their blood."

In the cheaper resorts that catered mostly to colored people, a wilder license prevailed. Samuel Hazard, whose excellent book *Cuba with Pen and Pencil* was published in 1871, refers discreetly to a ball watched in the assembly room of the Café Escauriza. The female partners at that popular spot were chiefly mulattoes, though he does not say so. "They are dancing their favorite Cuban dance, the *danza*," he writes, "pretty enough and proper enough when danced with fair women and proper men; but as danced here, one of the most indecent spectacles I have ever seen at any public ball." A Cuban contemporary, moreover, spoke of the "infernal chattering" of the music that never ceased for a moment, the "satyr-like delirium" of the movements in which the women assumed the active part and the men the passive.

The general profligacy was reflected in the fact that during the 1870's and 1880's the average of illegitimate births in the city of Havana ran to about 45 per cent. Yet there was ample scope for prostitution as well. Except for a short period under Tacón, the institution had been open and rampant; now it exceeded all bounds. One notes with astonishment that it had never even been regulated until the adoption of an ordinance on December 27, 1873, which served to encourage rather than to limit it. The police segregated the houses into five groups; the first comprised sixty-two houses, the second nineteen, the third seventeen, the fourth forty-six, and the fifth thirty. The larger divisions must have consisted of small buildings, for the number of occupants was recorded as being from eighty to a hundred in each group. The most thickly occupied street was Bomba, in Group One, where there were thirty-one houses.

Dr. Benjamin de Céspedes published his curious history,

La Prostitución en la Ciudad de la Habana, in 1888. His approach is coolly medical, but he has an eye for the picturesque. He writes that the display of prostitution in the 1880's was "more nude and shameless than even in the bazaars of Malta and eastern ports." The windows of the houses were kept open on fine nights, and the women could be seen posturing within. Also, the well-to-do professionals did not hesitate to go driving in their *quitríns* among the best society.

The author condemns the crowded stews of Bomba and of a stretch on Monserrate called the Recinto, paralleling the old walls. He advises that these two should be demolished as menaces to health. Apparently he had his way, for both names have disappeared, Bomba being widened and made into a westward extension of the Calle San Juan de Dios. But he speaks tolerantly of the houses in Group Five, on San Miguel, Consulado and Virtudes, as offering "refined prostitution" in Havana.

Dr. Céspedes tells some typical stories. Upon the death of a certain official in Havana, his friends gossiped freely about the man. His departmental superior, who was high in state councils in Madrid, had sent him to Cuba on promotion, and he had left behind his wife and daughter, hoping to make a quick fortune and rejoin them. But the superior had arranged the transfer because he was the wife's lover, according to the tale. No one knew whether to believe it. Confirmation was soon had. The wife and daughter appeared in Havana, the former alleging that their home existence had become precarious. After friends of her dead husband had given her a little help, it was learned that the patron in Madrid had cast her off and nobody would have anything more to do with her.

The daughter leapt into the breach, proving herself to be a born harlot. She accepted the attentions of an oldish merchant and looted his bank account. When he could stand her no longer she went on the town. Her earnings were very large and she was generous with her mother. But it was only her mother that she enriched. She herself had a mania for gambling and for buying clothes, jewels, and luxuries of all kinds. In a few years she had sunk from star cocotte to inmate of an ordinary bordello.

Then there was the daughter of a woman who had made a fortune in the Canary Islands by running a famous house much patronized between 1855 and 1862. A lover wasted the madame's money and ended by growing infatuated with the young daughter. So the latter was sent to a relative in Havana, with the frank design of getting her launched in a career of profitable harlotry. The first thing this damsel did was to auction her virginity for $200. The buyer made her his mistress for a while. On his abandoning her to return to Spain, she became a full prostitute and had uncommon success before she was overtaken by disease and premature old age.

"The white *bata*, which imitates fashionable negligée so well," writes Dr. Céspedes, "crimped at the swelling of the bosom by the superimposing of silk ribbons and bows combined, the lace kerchief, the silk stockings, the luxury costume for balls, for receptions, for the rumba; the slippers sown with golden butterflies, the shoes, the petticoat complicated with underskirts; the fashionable hard corset sheathed with black or bronze-colored satin, like a martial breastplate; the perfume, the rouge, the finger-ring, the ornaments for apparel and dressed hair, the knick-knacks—all these luxurious props have come to be for them [cocottes] as necessary as food, or as the very air they breathe." It is a period picture.

On the lowest level of the population, among the poorest blacks, there was *ñáñigo*, which should not be confused with the form of voodoo called *brujería francesa* in the eastern part of Cuba. *Náñigo*, too, was based upon primitive African religion, but its structure was that of linked secret societies comparable to masonic lodges. It was as old as slavery itself in the island.

At its best *ñáñigo* furnished a system of mutual aid among membership and brightened their lives with hilarious entertainment. The Dia de Los Reyes (Twelfth Night) was adopted by them as their chief public festival, when they pranced in bizarre costumes through the streets. At times they appeared, masked, in the carnival parades. That there was a criminal side to their activities cannot be denied. One Cuban authority of the last century states that "the *ñáñigos* form an association dark with robbery and violence." This was true enough during the Ten Years' War and the days that immediately followed it.

Chapter 16

THE WAR OF INDEPENDENCE

SUCH WAS the Havana to which José Julián Martí, benefiting by a general amnesty, returned in August, 1878. He had graduated brilliantly in law at the universities of Madrid and Saragossa, and though he intended to practice the profession the dominant impulse of his life had nothing to do with Spanish law. He had shown great gifts as a speaker and writer, and all his utterances had been in behalf of Cuba. He was convinced that the cause of independence was not lost, but had merely received a check. There had crystallized in him a decision to give all of himself to the rebuilding of the national effort on a basis so patriotically sound, so carefully planned, that it must succeed. Yet he cannot be said to have taken the first practical step in that direction prior to his arrival in Havana at the age of twenty-five years and seven months.

Martí had a grave and esthetic though not a puritanical nature. He was distressed by the corruption of life in the capital. He could better understand the deep scepticism and discouragement among politically minded men, regarding that as a sickness which would be shaken off. Martí entered the law office of a friend, the liberal Nicolás Azcárate, who one day introduced him to a young mulatto named Juan Gualberto Gómez. In the latter Martí found a genuine revolutionist with beliefs similar to his own, and they became close friends. Quickly they passed to actual, premature plotting.

Azcárate's office was not prosperous, and in a few months Martí was forced to change over to that of Miguel Viondi. He was given plenty of work there, but the likelihood of his making a financial success of it may be judged by the fact that he often scoffed at the law as a "deceitful profession." His oratory won praise. He came into demand at ceremonial and literary gatherings. When a chance arose, however, at a banquet held in honor of a publisher who favored sueing for concessions from Spain, Martí responded to a toast by saying firmly, "Rights are taken, not begged." He added: "If we are to constrain the heart so that truth may not surge from it by way of the lips . . . if we must wear masks, then I cover my glass; I do not toast Cuban politics." And he sat down without having drunk.

The new captain general was Ramón Blanco, who had succeeded Mártinez Campos after the war. He was told that the audience had applauded Martí's sentiments, and being a well-meaning man he took the first opportunity to go and hear the young Cuban speak instead of having him interrogated by the police. This time the subject was the work of a local violinist. There were many references to liberty and the national ideal, which Blanco shrugged aside with the remark that they had no great importance. He added that Martí seemed cracked to him and possibly dangerous. The measure of both men is to be found in the captain general's judgment: of José Martí whose divine madness created his country, and of Ramón Blanco the temporizer who would one day be sent back by Spain to wind up affairs.

Guerrilla forces raised the flag briefly in Santiago province. This encouraged the Havana conspirators, whose numbers increased steadily; they met every day in one private house or another, including Martí's home in the Calle Industria. Antonio Maceo sent an encouraging message from exile in Jamaica. But the secret service had become aware of them. Late in 1879 there was a raid that trapped all the leaders. No one was sentenced to death, but many were deported. Juan Gualberto Gómez drew confinement in a North African penal colony. Martí was simply exiled to Spain, but with the proviso that he must never set foot again in Cuba.

The course of Martí was now clear to himself, no matter who might think it visionary. He slipped out of Spain and landed in New York on January 3, 1880, where he joined the Cuban junta that had long been active but needed rejuvenation. Soon he was its directing spirit. The industry and oneness of purpose that he showed may have been equaled by other revolutionary leaders; it can never have been surpassed. He saw that he would have to depend largely upon Cubans living away from the island, some as political refugees, some as merchants and workmen. Martí had great natural talent as an organizer. He built up committees and clubs already existing in New York, Mexico City, and particularly in Tampa and Key West, Florida, where most of the hands in the cigar factories were Cubans. He later established many new groups among his countrymen wherever he could find them—in the eastern cities of the United States, in all the Latin American countries around the Caribbean Sea, and in Jamaica.

At almost the outset of this phase of his work, Martí was compelled to assist a minor insurrection in eastern Cuba which is known as the Little War. It was really a continuation of the Ten Years' War by men who had rejected the terms of surrender to the Spaniards. Martí did not believe in this effort, because he knew that the first essential was to organize. But he could not withhold his support from patriots such as Calixto García and José Maceo, who were resolved to fight. The Little War soon collapsed, as he had expected.

The Cuban military leaders were scattered in exile. Martí kept up a correspondence with Máximo Gómez and Antonio Maceo, in fact with all of them, telling them of his work, stimulating them to ardor for the next attempt. Most of them were older men than he, and they had to be wooed into accepting guidance from him. Without exception, they ended by admiring him wholeheartedly. A special title was conceded to him. He became the Apostle. It was to take fifteen long years for him to reach his objective—and his martyrdom.

A general impression of life in Havana during the earlier years of the fifteen was given in the preceding chapter. After Martí's influence from abroad began to be appreciated, a stiffening of morale took place among those citizens who loved their country. These were in the vast majority, though Spanish oppression silenced the voices of all but the boldest. Regular financial contributions to the New York junta were now made from Havana. Thousands of young men prepared themselves for service under arms by pistol and fencing practice. Discussion groups studied the principles of self-government as openly as they dared.

The sidewalk tables of the Louvre Café on the Prado facing the Parque Isabel (now Parque Central) constituted a rendezvous of political intellectuals, mostly young men of good families who were not afraid of getting into arguments with Spanish officers and, if necessary, seeing the matter through on the field of honor. The enemy were somewhat more suave than in the old days, more inclined to treat certain Cubans as equals.

Federico Villoch, in his *Viejas Postales Descoloridas (Old Faded Post Cards)*, tells that one evening in 1890 Antonio Maceo, though a banished outlaw, appeared at the Louvre, correctly dressed in a frock coat. He was accompanied by Agustín Cervantes, a valiant Cuban duelist, who introduced him to Brigadier General Fidel de Santocildes of the Spanish army. Santocildes, whose personality some young Cubans admired, discussed military matters amicably with Maceo and described the tactics he would use against him if he ever got the chance. The story is almost too good to be true, especially as five years later Santocildes died in the bush fighting Maceo; but I repeat it for what it is worth.

The Spaniards were well aware of the activities of Martí and other exiles, which after 1892 included gunrunning to Cuba. Reserves of arms and ammunition were being accumulated in the mountains. The early complaints to the United States government did not have much effect. Perhaps in the hope of gaining support, Spain agreed to a reciprocity treaty which had long been urged upon her and admitted North American goods to Cuba at a reduced customs tariff. Trade with the big neighbor at once boomed, greatly to the satisfaction of the Havana merchants. But Spain's stupidity was incurable. Without warning she canceled the treaty in 1894. This, on top of the world financial panic of 1893 which drove down the price of sugar, created unemployment in the island and a restlessness that was conducive to action. This, as much as any other cause, decided Martí that the moment to strike had come.

He was ready toward the end of 1894. But an expedition consisting of three ships was halted in Florida under the neutrality laws and very important supplies of munitions were seized. The enforced postponement lasted for weeks only, whereas the Spaniards had hoped for months. On February 24, 1895, the Cry of Baire launched the War of Independence at the village of that name in Santiago province.

Detractors had said that José Martí would ask his compatriots to die while he sat in an easy chair in New York. He concluded that it was necessary to disprove this sneer. He had never borne arms, but that was equally true of thousands who were volunteering. Over the objections of his associates on the junta and of most of the generals, he resolved to take part in the first campaign, though it was agreed that he would leave Cuba after he had demonstrated his courage. Coming from that self-sacrificing spirit, it was a gesture of humility.

Martí joined Máximo Gómez in the Dominican Republic. They traveled across Haiti, where they took ship. Accompanied by a few followers, they reached Cuba in an open boat that had been dropped from a freighter in the Windward Passage. A few weeks later, on May 19th, the small command ran into an ambush at Dos Rios. Gómez asked Martí to keep to the rear, using the expression, "for this is not your place." But Martí would have none of that. He joined in the charge and was shot dead in his first skirmish. His end so shocked and grieved the Cuban people that they rose to the support of the revolution with a fervor they might not otherwise have shown. Antonio Maceo, his brother José Maceo, Calixto García and all the other noted leaders from the Ten Years' War were in the field. New ones emerged. The struggle was to rage for longer than three years.

Havana never revolted, as patriots had hoped might be the case, but its fortunes and its sympathies were deeply involved. This time the war was carried from end to end of the island. Spain had rushed General Martínez Campos back to the scene of his triumph in 1878. He was no longer the man he had been, whereas Gómez and Maceo had improved greatly. They whipped him in engagement after engagement, and forced him to take refuge in the capital. Before the first year ended, Máximo Gómez had raided the Havana suburb of Marianao, while Antonio Maceo had swept Pinar del Rio, the most westerly province. Martínez Campos asked to be relieved.

The new captain general sent by Spain was the most sinister personality to rule Cuba since Tacón, whom he did not equal in statecraft but far surpassed in cruelty. He was General Valeriano Weyler, Marquis of Teneriffe, soon to be known as the "Butcher." Weyler was an undersized man, shriveled and acrid, who wore black side-whiskers and mustache that looked as if they were dyed. He walked with a hurried strut. His alien-sounding name derived from part German-Jewish ancestry. Weyler had been military attaché at the Spanish legation in Washington during the War of Secession. He had accompanied General William T. Sherman as observer on several campaigns and vastly admired Sherman's tactics, particularly on the march through Georgia. Later as a subordinate commander he had applied terroristic methods in Cuba during the Ten Years' War.

Weyler was given a free hand and enormous reinforcements of troops. The Spaniards in the field presently outnumbered the Cubans eight to one. The hyena-like *voluntarios* were increased by the recruiting of criminals from the jails and set at the throats of their fellow-countrymen, with license to practice whatever atrocities they chose. This corps of irregulars came to be known as *guerrilleros*, while the patriots were the *Mambís*, a term that had first come into use in the previous war. Free Cuba outside the cities was the *manigua*, or bush. When Weyler found that he could not win battles he adopted his most notorious measure, the reconcentration camps. Women and children, as well as males who had not taken up arms, were ordered into garrisoned towns and herded behind barbed wire. The deaths of these unfortunates from starvation and disease reached horrifying figures. The execution of prisoners in the Ditch of the Laurels at the Cabaña fortress, Havana, was an almost daily event.

In December, 1896, Antonio Maceo fell in an ambush at Punta Brava in Havana province, and with him died the young Francisco Gómez, son of the Generalissimo. It was a hard blow for Cuba. Weyler, exultant, praised Maceo as a "valiant man, a fighter, indefatigable, tenacious," scoffed at Gómez as being too old and sick to carry on alone, and predicted a quick end to the revolution. He was mistaken.

Máximo Gómez in his grief proved more effective than ever. And Weyler's own barbarities had turned public opinion in the United States against Spain. The New York junta, now headed by Tomás Estrada Palma, received generous gifts from American sympathizers. Under veiled pressure from Washington, the administration in Madrid removed Weyler late in 1897 and Ramón Blanco, the man from the past, replaced him. A fairly liberal form of self-government was proclaimed for Cuba. Gómez would have none of it. He declared that any Cuban who subscribed to Spain's brand of autonomy was a traitor and he executed at least one man who had the temerity to approach him as a mediator. With the exception of a few defeatists in the capital, the Cubans applauded him. The war went on.

Havana was destined, after all, to be the scene of the most sensational event of the crisis. On January 25, 1898, the U.S.S. *Maine* arrived in port on what was termed a "courtesy call," but actually to observe conditions affecting American citizens. The Spaniards were outwardly polite. They designated the spot where the ship must anchor. Visits were exchanged by her commander and Captain General Blanco. Three weeks later, on the night of February 15th, the *Maine* was wrecked by a mysterious explosion and foundered with a loss of 260 officers and men. Intense excitement prevailed in the city. Blanco sent condolences and apparently did his best to arrive at the truth of what had happened. Then and afterward it was reasonably clear that some exterior force, presumably a mine, had destroyed the armored cruiser. The harbor was sown with mines, which were not of the contact type, but controlled by wires from a point on the shore. The identity of the individual, perhaps a Spaniard, perhaps a Cuban, who touched off the explosion has never been established.

The United States was in the mood to condemn Spain —and Spain only—for a crowning outrage, and on April 25th war was declared. A close naval blockade of Havana caused material hardships in the city. Fighting, however, was confined to the east, around Santiago de Cuba, where Admiral Pascual Cervera's ships were sunk by the American fleet under Commodore Winfield S. Schley, and the Spanish land forces crushed at San Juan Hill and El Caney by

General W. R. Shafter's army, effectively aided by Cuban troops under General Calixto García. Theodore Roosevelt led his regiment, the Rough Riders, at San Juan Hill. This is not the place to retell the well-known story of the short, sharp struggle which figures in United States annals as the Spanish-American War, but which island historians prefer to call the Spanish-Cuban-American War.

Spain capitulated in August. She signed the treaty under which she gave up Cuba in December. On January 1, 1899, the one hundred and thirty-sixth and last governor sailed with the last Spanish troops from Havana, and the same day a United States army of occupation took over the city.

Chapter 17

TUTELAGE BY THE U.S.A.

CUBAN AUTHORITIES believe that unaided their forces would eventually have triumphed. I accept this view, for the double reason that Spanish losses from yellow fever had been fantastically high and that after the failure of Weyler's terroristic methods Spanish morale declined. The military genius of Gómez is, of course, a third and excellent reason. Gómez had asked the United States to fight the enemy only at sea and cut off their supplies from Europe, while he attended to their armies. The idea had been overruled, and it is obvious that victory was won much more speedily by the

direct intervention in the east. But the American decision
to administer the island until it had been educated in the
ways of self-government was painful to Cubans. They
showed considerable restraint when they accepted the period of tutelage instead of staying under arms. For there
was a school of political thought in the United States which
openly advocated the breaking of promises and the annex-
ing of Cuba.

General John R. Brooke was appointed military governor
and took over the palace of the captains general in Havana.
He found the city physically dirty beyond words and its
public buildings gutted. The evacuating Spaniards had ma-
liciously left chaos behind them. They had broken up the
plumbing and lighting fixtures, had choked the very drains
with refuse. Everything that could be removed had been
stolen. The customs house had been stripped bare of furniture, its records destroyed. Not a single stamp or piece
of small change could be discovered in the post office.

It was not until February 24, 1899, that Generalissimo
Máximo Gómez entered Havana at the head of a Mambí
brigade. The date had been chosen because it was the anniversary of the Cry of Baire that had started the War of
Independence. He was given a delirious welcome. As Be-
nigno Souza, one of his biographers, puts it: "The glorious
little old man was literally unable to take a step for many
days without finding himself overwhelmed by the kisses and
embraces of the women, from the most haughty down
to the most humble workwoman; and his residence, the
Quinta de los Molinos, summer palace of the Spanish captains general, was the rendezvous of all who meant something then in Cuba." Here was evidence, if any were
needed, of the true sentiments of the people.

But Gómez was an austere patriot, and he was soon
under fire from selfish elements. An assembly of delegates

from the Cuban army had been in existence since early in
the war. The United States authorities welcomed the views
of this assembly, but were not bound by them. New York
financial interests offered to lend Cuba a large sum. The
local politicians were eager that it should be accepted, and
General Brooke might have agreed if the support of Gómez
could have been obtained. When the old Generalissimo
learned that the terms of the loan would be at 38 per cent
discount, he emphatically denounced the whole scheme and
it fell through. Also, he consented on realistic grounds to
disband the Cuban forces upon the distribution of $3,000,-
000 as an outright gift from the United States, which
worked out at some seventy-five dollars to each soldier. No
larger grant could have been obtained. It had been hoped,
however, to divide up $60,000,000 from the proposed loan
and other sources, which Gómez scotched.

For the above reasons, the Assembly actually voted to
remove Máximo Gómez as commander-in-chief. An immense popular demonstration in his honor immediately
resulted. Veterans, ordinary citizens, and students from the
university marched cheering to the Quinta de los Molinos
for three days in succession. Gómez was pleased, but he
insisted on moving to the very modest home of a friend in
Havana, remarking: "If they want to get rid of me alto-
gether, I have four other flags I can claim." He meant that
he was a native of the Dominican Republic, had lived as
a refugee in Jamaica, Honduras, and the United States, and
had had children born in all four countries. Washington
had not recognized the demotion of Gómez. The Assembly
dissolved itself in the face of the clamor it had caused.
Smiling cryptically, the old man returned to the Quinta de
los Molinos, his influence enhanced.

He detested city life and intrigues, all the same. "You
don't know the infamies of this Havana. Never come to

live here," he wrote to a woman friend at the time. "I do not wish to hear a word about politics, and of the nastiness of this place, much less!"

Brooke made a beginning with sanitation, the creating of government departments in which Cubans were given many offices, the raising of revenue, and schools. He was a well-meaning man but none too effective. Before the end of the year he was replaced by General Leonard Wood, the friend of Theodore Roosevelt. He had fought at San Juan Hill and had been made the first American provincial governor of Santiago. Wood's energy was great, his judgment of problems sound, and his grasp of local psychology moderately good. He was inclined to be dictatorial, and this ruffled the Cubans, but no one questioned his honesty. All that Brooke had attempted he improved upon and more besides. The police, the courts, the hospitals, were brought to a high level of efficiency never approached under the Spaniards.

Public health was a major concern with Leonard Wood. He had had to deal with a yellow fever epidemic in Santiago, and it had puzzled him. No one understood yellow fever. It was thought to be a disease generated in dirty surroundings, and to be contagious as well as infectious. Wood resolved that he would make it impossible in Havana. He ordered his chief sanitation officer, Major William C. Gorgas, to clean the city thoroughly, and it was done. Yet the fever appeared afterward, in the hot months of 1900. Wood had the insight to conclude that the old theories must be wrong. So he appointed a military commission headed by Dr. Walter Reed, with Drs. James Carroll, Jesse W. Lazear, and Aristides Agramonte. The orders were to test and experiment until every possibility was exhausted.

Dr. Carlos Finlay, a Cuban physician of Scots ancestry,

had told the Academy of Sciences, Havana, twenty years before that mosquitoes conveyed yellow fever from man to man. He believed that a single species, the *stegomyia*, was responsible, but he did not know in just what circumstances. Finlay took this theory to the commission, and it was tried out after other approaches had proved fruitless. The result was a victory in 1901, which I appraise in my history, *The Caribbean*, as being a greater one by far than any that has terminated a war between nations. I repeat that assertion.

United States soldiers volunteered as guinea pigs at Quemados, a special camp near Havana. They were exposed under varied conditions: They slept in beds where yellow-fever patients had died, wore clothing taken from corpses, were left unprotected from mosquitoes which had bitten sufferers—in clean beds as well as foul ones. No one caught the disease if his room had been properly screened against the insects. Many who were stung got it, and some of them died. Before the principle had been completely established, Drs. Carroll and Lazear of the commission caused themselves to be bitten. Both of them developed yellow fever. Carroll barely recovered and Lazear died.

At last it was known for certain that the female *stegomyia* transmitted the malady, that she incubated the germ only if she had sucked the blood of a patient within the first three days of his illness, and that she could pass it on only after a delay of from twelve to twenty days. The male was harmless. Armed with this knowledge, Major Gorgas extirpated the mosquitoes of Havana by fumigating with sulphur to get those on the wing and treating the surface of stagnant water with oil to destroy the unhatched larvae. The scourge vanished from the city. In due course the method was applied throughout the American tropics, and notably on the Isthmus of Panama as a preliminary to the digging of the canal. Dr. Finlay deserves full honor in history along with the devoted men who proved the value of his idea.

As might be expected, the American administration was rather straitlaced. It outlawed the bullfight as a matter of course, and Cubans approved of that. But it also put a ban upon cockfighting, which led to much bad humor among ordinary citizens. The lottery was abolished and a campaign was waged against gambling. Wood, however, granted a concession for the game of *jai-alai*. That cocks were fought and money risked in a dozen ways behind the scenes cannot be doubted. The sum total of naughtiness may have been reduced. Anyhow, the public aspect of the cocking main and the noisy placing of bets meant more than half the fun to the people. No serious attempt was made to end prostitution, which at that time ran wide open in most cities of the United States.

Two important physical changes wrought in the capital by Wood were the reconstruction of the Prado and the laying out of the Malecón. It will be remembered that the first-mentioned promenade had been beautified by Tacón, who had called it the Paseo de Isabel II, a name which was now dropped. Wood widened it and paved the central walk, planted a double row of laurel trees to shade it, and improved the driveways on both sides. He must be given the major credit for the Malecón, though the plan was first suggested by General de Albear, a Cuban engineer, in 1857. The curving waterfront of Havana running westward along the ocean had been left as a rocky shoreline with a narrow street on top of it. Wood created the finest boulevard of its sort in the West Indies, protected for miles by an embankment.

There was a good deal of less inspired construction work by individuals. American business interests had flocked into

Havana, bought sites cheap and replaced fine houses with the ugly office buildings of the period. Even the narrowest colonial streets, such as Obispo and O'Reilly, were not spared. The palaces that remain in Old Havana escaped by luck, or because of the fact that they were still occupied by well-to-do families who did not need to sell.

Governor Wood had been instructed by Washington to prepare Cuba for independence as a republic. Both President McKinley and his successor Roosevelt were sincere about this; they had resisted the machinations of the powerful groups in the United States which wanted the island annexed. Wood held municipal elections in the summer of 1900, and Havana installed its first mayor under the new order. Then delegates were chosen to a convention that wrote Cuba's constitution. A document setting forth future relations between the two countries was drafted and most of it embodied in the constitution under North American pressure. The United States got the naval base at Guantánamo Bay outright and retained an ambiguous stake in the Isle of Pines. The Platt Amendment limited the foreign relations and the public debt of Cuba and provided that the United States "might intervene for the preservation of Cuban independence, the maintenance of a government adequate for the protection of life, property, and individual liberty," et cetera.

All this made Cuba a sort of protectorate rather than a fully independent country and was found humiliating. Nevertheless, the terms were accepted.

A presidential election was called for December 31, 1901. Political parties had naturally been formed before then. The majority faction wanted Máximo Gómez as its candidate, and he could almost certainly have been elected. A clause had been added to the constitution to make him eligible, since he was of foreign birth. But the doughty veteran declined with a memorable phrase: "Men of war, for war; and those of peace, for peace." Later he said, with shrewd mockery, to friends who urged him vainly to reconsider: "Perhaps I fear the vertigo that seizes one at great heights."

Gómez offered his support to Tomás Estrada Palma. An opposition party nominated General Bartolomé Masó, the last provisional president in the *manigua*, but decided after all not to go to the polls. The head of the New York junta, who did not even return to Cuba to campaign, was allowed to have a clean sweep.

The Americans set May 20, 1902, as the day for turning over Cuba to her own officials. There seems to have been no particular reason for the choice, except departmental convenience. May 19th would have been more appropriate, for that was the anniversary of the death of José Martí. But the citizens of Havana, frenzied with joy, were not in the mood to cavil. The letting off of skyrockets from the Cabaña fortress began at sunset on the 19th and continued until dawn. The cafés stayed open all night. Crowds danced on the Prado, on most of the great central streets, and in the parks. They massed the next day in front of the palace of the captains general, and at the foot of the Prado commanding the best view of Morro Castle. For at noon the flag of the single star was raised on the palace, and a few minutes later on the Morro.

General Wood formally relinquished office to Estrada Palma, who was sworn in. It was Cuba Libre at last.

Chapter 18

UNDER THE EARLY PRESIDENTS

Tomás Estrada Palma was the most virtuous, honest man ever to serve as President of Cuba. His habits were simple; he did not care at first to live in the palace of the captains general, but would ride there in the morning on a street car and chat with anybody who addressed him. He carried forward all vital public works, but had a passion for economy and accumulated a large surplus in the treasury. A standing army was abhorrent to him, and he budgeted only for rural guards. Far stricter morally than Leonard Wood, he vetoed a lottery act, with a horrified reference to an attempt that had been made to restore the cockfight.

Life in Havana during his first four years was consequently dull. It may seriously be questioned whether his extreme goodness was the best medicine for the young republic. Cuba's temperament ran contrary to his. A fighting hero of the revolution would certainly have aroused more enthusiasm and might not have brewed discord. As it was, the very economy of Estrada Palma caused trouble, and his lack of an army encouraged the malcontents. One cannot help wondering how the great José Martí would have fared as president. He, too, was austere and pure.

There was no bar in the constitution to a second term. But it had been assumed that Estrada Palma, who had been sixty-seven when he took office, would not run again. Máximo Gómez did not think that he should and gave his support to the candidacy of General Emilio Núñez. Then in June, 1905, the Generalissimo died and the chances of Núñez evaporated. The Liberal Party was formed. It nominated the ebullient General José Miguel Gómez, not related to the Generalissimo, but a lieutenant who had distinguished himself in the field and was now the political boss of Santa Clara province. The friends of Estrada Palma shouted that the chief aim of the Liberals was to loot the treasury, where there was a balance of about $25,000,000, and that only the president himself could prevent that scandal. He must take a second term. It was an argument calculated to move him. He got to believe it himself, and reluctantly he accepted the nomination.

The upshot was tragic. His worst enemy never supposed that Don Tomás ordered the ballot boxes to be stuffed. It remains a fact that he naively allowed his supporters to conduct affairs in the way they saw fit, and the election proved as corrupt as it well could be. He was inaugurated for the second time under a cloud. Three months later, elements that had favored Gómez broke out in sporadic revolts all over the island. Disillusioned, the president resigned and asked the United States to act under the terms of the Platt Amendment.

Most Cubans feel to this day that he did the wrong thing. Several compromises had been suggested. President Theodore Roosevelt sent Secretary of War William Howard Taft to Havana as a mediator and declared that he hoped not to have to intervene. Estrada Palma stubbornly walked out to an old age of dignified poverty in Santiago de Cuba. Taft ruled for two weeks. Then Roosevelt appointed Charles E. Magoon governor, and governor he remained for two years and three months.

This was not at all what the rebellious faction had anticipated. It had thought there would be a brief occupation and the holding of new elections. American mercantile interests rejoiced, however, and so did many Havana businessmen. The United States consul, Frank Steinhardt, an ex-soldier, resigned presently and grew rich as a promoter. The Magoon regime, in spite of good intentions, became an unfortunate episode.

Paradoxically, Magoon was as honest an individual in money matters as Don Tomás, but he was not economical and he was easily fooled. The Liberals swarmed about him, posing as the injured party in whose behalf the intervention had been necessary, and he soothed them with jobs that too often were sinecures. He pardoned criminals wholesale. He handed out contracts for public works in reckless fashion, favoring his own countrymen above natives. The surplus in the treasury vanished with amazing rapidity, but evidence that Magoon pocketed any of it has not been adduced.

Cubans disliked the portly and lethargic governor who had no bonhomie. Liberals and Conservatives finally joined in denouncing him. Enrique Barbarossa called him, "A star without light." Miguel Lozano Casado wrote unfairly: "Gross in type, rude of manners—he falls like a buzzard on the Cuban treasury and devours it." Magoon did nothing whatsoever to improve the city of Havana. He did take a census which showed that the population had risen to 302,526.

In 1908 Washington announced presidential elections, to be held on November 14th, and the parties indulged in frantic maneuvers. José Miguel Gómez again headed the Liberals, and Alfredo Zayas who had sought to displace him was chosen as his running mate. Young General Mario G. Menocal was nominated by the Conservatives, inheriting the following of Tomás Estrada Palma. It had been made clear that the election must be peaceful, or the intervention would not end. So it was conducted honestly. The Liberals adopted as their emblem a cock perched on a plough which signified, they declared, "vigilance and industry." But to the common people in town and country it meant a promise to legalize cockfighting once more. Gómez made no bones about saying on the stump that he would be a real "liberal" when it came to popular amusements. This had irresistible appeal, and he won by a large majority.

Magoon turned the government over to Gómez on January 28, 1909, and sailed away, less than regretted. A bill to restore the cockfight was at once rushed through the Cuban Congress. It was followed by a lottery law and other legislation designed to create a free-and-easy atmosphere. Opponents called it going back to the evil ways of the Spaniards. The logical counter-arguments were heard, that Cubans were indeed Spanish Americans and not Anglo-Saxon Americans, that they saw no sin in gambling, that the cockfight was a local variation of sport. Had they not rejected the bullfight, which was typically Spanish and bad?

Gómez became immensely popular in Havana, as he had long been in his native Santa Clara. He kept magnificent open house, loved good-fellowship, gambling, and all recreations. "I have ever been jovial in spirits, a smile on my lips," he said of himself. Being a cattle rancher, part of his pose was to dress in rough-seeming but costly clothes, with silver spurs, and a broad-brimmed Panama hat. He fancied the girls. It was well understood that he grafted to pay for his fun and to lay by a nest egg. It happened to be a prosperous period, and few criticized him. He was even given the nickname of *El Tiburón*, "the Shark," as a term of affection.

I have been told that every would-be concessionaire, if

big enough, would at last find himself alone with Gómez in his office. All the facts had been furnished the president, of course. He would say genially, "Have a cigar!" push a box toward the man and then turn to look out of the window. The box contained a few cigars and some money as a silent hint. When Gómez turned back, he would glance to see whether a generous sum had been added and decide the case accordingly. Those were simple times.

Provision for an army of 5,000 men had been made under Magoon, and it was zestfully established by Gómez. He had come out strongly for the principle of a single term for presidents, but as his own drew to a close he obviously planned to use the army to win a second election. Things went awry and Zayas, his vice-president, was nominated. Gómez did not take this philosophically. He avenged himself by supporting Menocal, who was again the Conservative candidate, and the latter was elected.

Mario García Menocal took office with every advantage of personality, training, and prestige on his side. He was a cosmopolitan, having been educated in the United States as an engineer and employed for years on the project to dig an interoceanic canal in Nicaragua. He enlisted as a private when the War of Independence started, was soon commissioned and served under Máximo Gómez, Antonio Maceo and Calixto García in succession, rising to the rank of major general. He greatly distinguished himself at the action of Victoria de las Tunas. The United States military authorities appointed him chief of police of Havana. Turning to the sugar business, he made the Chaparra plantation the largest and best in the world. Influential North Americans believed in him. His name was known and respected in Europe. His own people esteemed him as a fine gentleman and patriot.

Yet Menocal's tenure of the presidency, which was to

last for eight years, can only be described as a strange patchwork of good and bad. He encouraged foreign investors more intelligently and honestly than his exuberant predecessor had done. Menocal did not rob the state himself. At the same time he allowed his partisans considerable freedom to make money on the side, and he had a failing that he indulged to a fantastic degree. He was a nepotist par excellence. Family connections, distant as well as close, were given jobs and were protected if they misbehaved. The taxpayers learned to their cost that there had never been so large a Cuban family as the Menocals, or one so lustful for office.

World War I caused financial difficulties in 1914. Barely a year later the price of sugar began to go up; when the United States entered the war it soared; and after the close of hostilities it reached an unprecedented figure. Cuba rolled in wealth. The boom was called the "Dance of the Millions." Menocal used some of the state's vast tax income to build a new presidential palace that suited his luxurious tastes, abandoning a smaller structure that had been started by Gómez.

In 1916 the president had contrived his re-election, defeating Zayas by means fully as irregular as those of Estrada Palma's supporters in 1906. Again the Liberals had flown to arms. But Menocal had an army. He swiftly crushed his enemies by a personal display of military talent, and thus averted another American intervention. The next four years were marked by an increase in cynicism. Menocal sat out the Dance of the Millions, only to see a financial crash in 1920 as sugar fell from twenty-two and a half cents to three and five-eighths cents a pound. He then arranged for his succession in a most unbecoming manner.

The Conservative nomination had been promised to General Núñez. Menocal concluded that he did not like this. He took over Alfredo Zayas, the perpetual Liberal aspirant, and ran him as a Conservative against José Miguel Gómez who was heading the Liberal ticket. This despite the fact that in 1912 Gómez had helped Menocal defeat Zayas. The 1920 struggle was not a democratic election. Bullying and brawling marked it, votes were stolen, and at the finish the retiring *caudillo* had his way. Dr. Zayas was installed as the fourth president of Cuba in May, 1921. Bitterly chagrined, José Miguel went to New York, where he got pneumonia in a few weeks and died. His funeral procession to the Colón Cemetery was the longest that had yet been seen in Havana.

Art and esthetics had their share of attention, as the Menocal regime merged into that of Zayas. Enrico Caruso attracted great audiences during his only engagement in the capital. Cuba glowed with pride when her son José Raúl Capablanca defeated Emmanuel Lasker in Havana, in 1921, for the chess championship of the world. The post of inspector of Cuban consulates was created for Capablanca, so that he could attend tournaments anywhere at the expense of the state.

That, also, was the date when Joseph Hergesheimer became infatuated with the city as a "mid-Victorian Pompeii" and wrote the most charming book about it that has ever been written in English, *San Cristóbal de la Habana*.

A noncombatant agitator in the War of Independence, a tricky lawyer and a morbid sensualist, Zayas was nicknamed *El Chino* because of his mask-like shaven countenance and his supposed Chinese patience. General Enoch Crowder had been forced on him by the United States to suggest reforms as a preliminary to the floating of a large loan. Zayas behaved fairly well until he had got rid of his mentor, and then he proceeded in two years to outdo all rivals as a grafter. They called him the "peseta stealer," the idea being that while José Miguel and others had lined their pockets with pesos (dollars), he did not let even the small change elude him. He made his son the director-general of the lottery and is said to have had at least one drawing manipulated to the benefit of his family. The Santa Clara Convent in Havana was bought for public purposes, the gigantic price of $2,350,000 being paid; the graft involved is believed to have been more than a million. Several lesser deals of the kind were put through. The palace drew revenue from protected gambling houses and agencies that were allowed to land prohibited Orientals in Cuba.

Zayas's only memorable effort to beautify the city was made after he learned that he would not be given a renomination. He thereupon appropriated $35,000 by decree to clear the ground behind the palace as a public square; it was to be landscaped, called Zayas Park and used as the setting for a statue of himself. Politicians and others who had profited by his rule received hints that they should subscribe to the monument fund, and they responded lavishly. Protests at his impudence were heard, but Zayas ignored them. Four days before the close of his term he had the statue unveiled. An inscription on its base avers that it was erected by a "grateful people" to the "restorer of the liberties of his country." The apologists for Zayas say that at least it was true that he never sought to overrule the Congress or interfered with private liberties.

His had obviously been the most evil presidency to date, but there was worse to come.

Chapter 19

MACHADO'S TYRANNY AND FALL

FORMER Spanish colonies in the New World have in
no single instance been able to enjoy a republican form of
government tranquilly from the start. We may ascribe this
to the vicious policies of Spain, which denied colonials
even the most elementary training in conducting their own
affairs, and endeavored, as far as possible, to keep them
ignorant of the workings of democracy in other countries.
The sad result has been that the revolution which won
liberty from Spain could not be the only one. Always there
has been violence later, to purge the state of evils inflicted
by robbers and despots. We have seen that Cuba had small
reason to be satisfied with her early presidents. But they
could be accepted in the hope that the public was learning
from them how to distinguish between the good and the
bad.

The island now had to face a tragic ordeal. Excess of
some sort had become probable. The emergence, however,
of one of the two or three most cruel dictatorships in the
history of Spanish America was not inevitable. It was a mis-
fortune. The fault lay with a monster, a scourge of God,
whom it would have been hard to appraise correctly before
he came to power, and who then rallied the support of
parasites and paid thugs.

132

General Gerardo Machado had been a brave fighter in the War of Independence, a founder of the Liberal Party, a cabinet minister under Gómez, and then a prominent merchant in the city of Santa Clara. He had been out of politics for seven years when he won the Liberal nomination over Colonel Carlos Mendieta, a better-known man, in 1924. The Conservatives had put up Menocal again, but the stench of the Zayas administration was so great that there was no chance for any but a Liberal that year. Machado was swept in, and for the first time in the history of Cuban elections the loser admitted his defeat and wrote a letter of congratulation.

All this pleased North American opinion. Possibly it influenced the United States Senate to ratify a treaty that canceled the claim to the Isle of Pines, which in turn made Cubans happy about the inauguration of Machado. His standing abroad and at home resembled that of Menocal in 1912. Nor did he begin badly. He put through a number of constructive measures, announced that he would build a central highway from end to end of Cuba and a splendid capitol in Havana, arranged for seemingly beneficial enterprises by foreigners. He did not seek loans in the United States until the start of 1927. Then the Chase National Bank and the house of Morgan, New York, tumbled over each other to risk money on so solid a customer.

Later that year, barely twenty-five months after he had taken office, Gerardo Machado showed his hand. He required Congress to pass amendments to the constitution which increased the presidential term to six years, added new senators and representatives, and established conditions that would make it impossible for any candidate to oppose the palace ticket in 1928. This was confirmed by a dazed constitutional convention that sat hedged metaphorically with bayonets. After going through the motions of an election, Machado reinstalled himself ostensibly until 1935.

Anger had flared against him from the moment he had asked for a change in the constitution. He had retorted by having many of his critics arrested, and it was hardly a matter for surprise that a few of them were never seen again. The strong political leaders outside his camp held their breath and counted their resources, aware that it was a case of acting vigorously or not at all. Students at the University of Havana protested openly, and the institution was closed off and on.

So far, it had been a typical Spanish American despotism. But as the opposition to him hardened, Machado's megalomania, cruelty, and greed swelled to inhuman proportions, and he appeared suddenly to go mad. One would not be far wrong in picking May 20, 1929, when his second term started, as the fatal date. It was widely believed in Cuba that about that time he developed the symptoms of paresis, the result of a venereal infection in early life. Along with his inauguration he celebrated the completion of the National Capitol, for which $3,500,000 had been originally authorized and which ended by costing nearly $20,000,000, more than half of it graft. He vaunted his central highway, a useful road indeed, but which was to absorb thousands of dollars per mile in excess of any similar thoroughfare on record. He slobbered over his friends and vowed vengeance on his foes.

A few weeks earlier the exiled student, Julio Antonio Mella, a young man of exceptional gifts, had been assassinated in Mexico City. No one doubted that Machado had had it done. Other manifesting students were now murdered in the streets of Havana; scores were imprisoned and the first rumors of torture were heard. Three hundred professors met openly and swore to support the youngsters of both sexes in their fight for a free government. Machado's answer was to nail planks across the doors of the university like a disused factory and post sentries on guard. Shortly afterward he closed the high schools and normal schools as well.

I have made the point in previous chapters that Havana did not play an active part in the conflicts with Spain. The capital's opportunity came in the struggle against Machado, and it lived up to it nobly. As a redeeming measure, this revolution was fully as necessary as the Ten Years' War and the War of Independence had been. It centered in Havana, was for the most part fought out in Havana.

The dictator formed his notorious Porra, or special police, and loosed it upon the people. There was an orgy of sadism that included the emasculation of youths and the ripping of women's breasts with gloves tipped with steel claws. Massacres were a commonplace, notably in the Cabaña fortress, where Spaniards had once butchered Cuban patriots, but where none could have anticipated that a president would ever slay his countrymen. Some victims were tossed to the sharks from the dungeons of Morro Castle. In the common jail at Príncipe Castle seventy political prisoners in a long gallery were dispatched with knives and blackjacks in a single coup.

Former President Menocal threw down the gage in a full-dress insurrection in August, 1931, accompanied by the landing of volunteers and supplies from the United States. It failed and he was captured, but the episode restored his glory as a national hero. Even Machado did not dare to harm so eminent a man. Menocal was allowed to go into exile, joining scores of distinguished Cubans and hundreds of ordinary refugees who had fled to save their lives. As in Martí's day, a New York junta functioned; its outposts were Miami in Florida, and Mérida in Yucatán.

The most vital development was the founding of the secret society called the ABC. Its membership was drawn chiefly from the intellectual and professional classes, was predominantly youthful, and comprised most of the militant students and teachers from the university. Dr. Ramón Grau San Martín, a physician and lecturer on anatomy, was among the leaders. In the savage irregular warfare that followed, many men and women of the greatest promise were killed, while new talents emerged. Grau was detected and jailed along with Dr. Carlos Finlay, son of the scientist who had discovered how yellow fever was transmitted. One day in 1932 the secret police arrested the young Eduardo Chibás and Carlos Prío Socarras. They were charged with capital crimes. Both escaped, to become important figures in the next phase of the republic.

Unemployment and low prices for Cuban products, the result of world-wide depression, added to the miseries of the people. But Machado continued to ride roughshod. When his friend Vásquez Bello, president of the Senate, was assassinated, he promptly had a score of Liberals butchered, including the three Freyre de Andrade brothers, whose father had been an eminent figure. Miguel Mariano Gómez, son of the second president, then serving as mayor of Havana, was driven from the country for condemning the wholesale reprisals.

Help came with the accession of Franklin D. Roosevelt to the presidency of the United States. There was no talk of armed intervention. Roosevelt, however, showed his abhorrence of the Machado tyranny by sending Sumner Welles as ambassador, under instructions to exert moral pressure. This meant much, for Cuba was still a protectorate. The ABC redoubled its efforts and hundreds of new members joined it. Machado made slight concessions to Welles, chiefly by setting free a number of political prisoners and relaxing the censorship of the press. He refused absolutely to resign.

On August 4, 1933, a transportation strike that appears not to have been closely connected with the revolution stung Machado into threatening to declare martial law and a state of war unless the men at once returned to work. This caused a sympathetic general strike which was backed by the ABC. For three days the life of the city was paralyzed. On the afternoon of August 7th, a voice proclaimed over the radio that Machado had been overthrown. Thousands believed it and started a parade to the palace. As they converged from the Prado and Zulueta, the police opened fire upon them with machine guns, killing 28 and wounding about 150. The radio announcement had been a fake on the part of the government, to give it an excuse for massacre. During the next few days the Porra swarmed through the streets, killing for sport.

This time Machado had gone too far. The army, on which his power rested, decided that it must co-operate with Ambassador Welles. The "Beast," as he had long been called, was deposed by officers. He got off easily, for they allowed him to escape by plane, carrying a suitcase filled with gold, to die a dog's death of his maladies some five years later in Miami.

It would have been too much to expect moderation of the Havana mob. The palace was partly sacked. The homes of many Machado supporters were looted and put to the torch. Such gestures did not suffice. There was a darker reckoning to be had with the police, for never in all history could policemen have been hated more intensely. The vile Antonio Jimínez, chief of the Porra, was recognized at the crossing of the Prado and Virtudes, shot to death and the corpse kicked about the street. Brigadier Antonio B. Ainciart, the sadistic chief of police, hid out for a while, and then was discovered masquerading as an old woman. He committed suicide. Major Arsenio Ortiz, perhaps the worst of the three, chief of the military police, had seen what was coming and had left Cuba.

Meanwhile, the leaders of the ABC, the students' organization, and the army had chosen as provisional president of the republic Dr. Carlos Manuel de Céspedes, son and namesake of the great patriot who had been the first provisional president in the Ten Years' War. The younger Céspedes had proved himself a gifted diplomat. He had been ambassador in Washington, Madrid, and Mexico. As a psychological choice he seemed perfect.

Chapter 20

THE SECOND PHASE OF THE REPUBLIC

THOUGH MANY problems remained and no subsequent administration has fully solved them, it can be said that with the fall of Machado a new phase began for the republic. At last it was mature. There has been dictatorship, but it has had to take account of the desires of the people. The progress toward honest elections has been steady, and an attempt to reverse it would not be tolerated. Graft persists, an evil by no means confined to Cuba, but a brazen attitude about it is no longer condoned.

Despite his glamorous name, Carlos Manuel de Céspedes

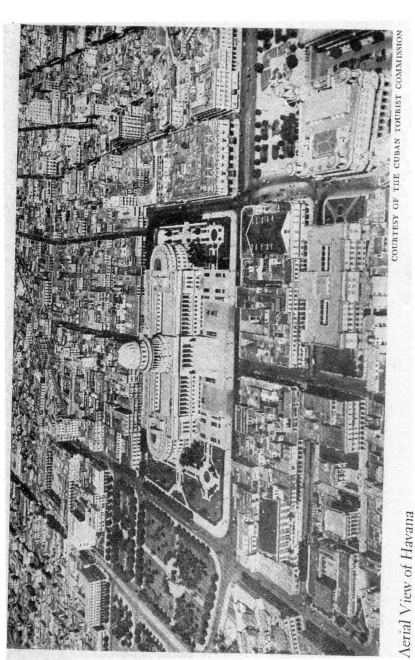

Aerial View of Havana

Havana

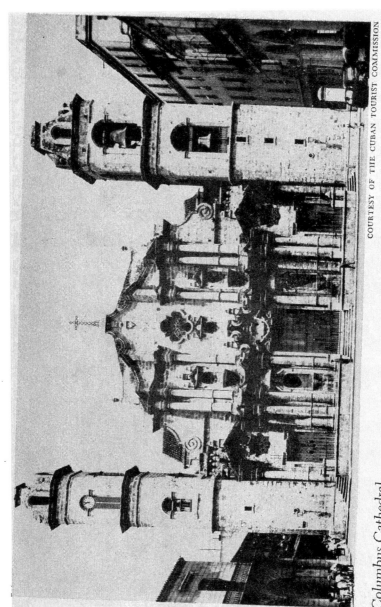

Columbus Cathedral

COURTESY OF THE CUBAN TOURIST COMMISSION

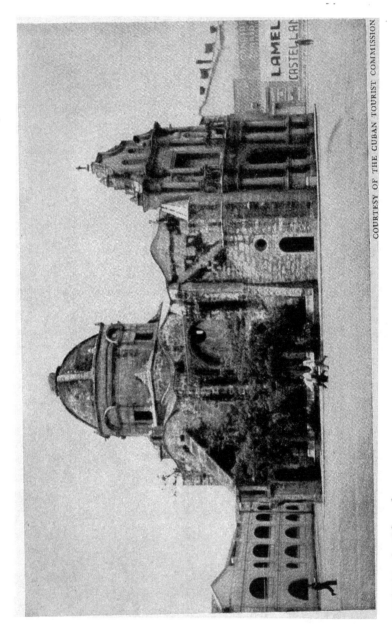

Old Paula Church

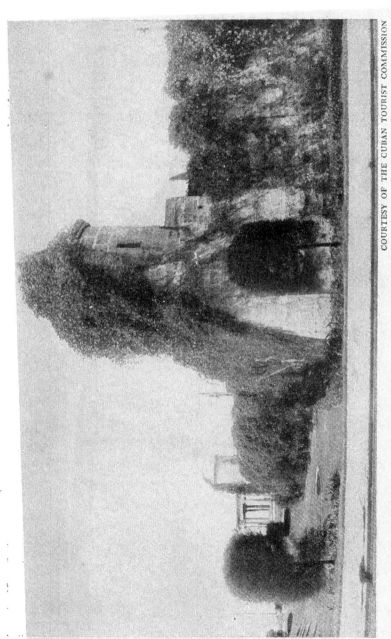

COURTESY OF THE CUBAN TOURIST COMMISSION

La Punta Fortress

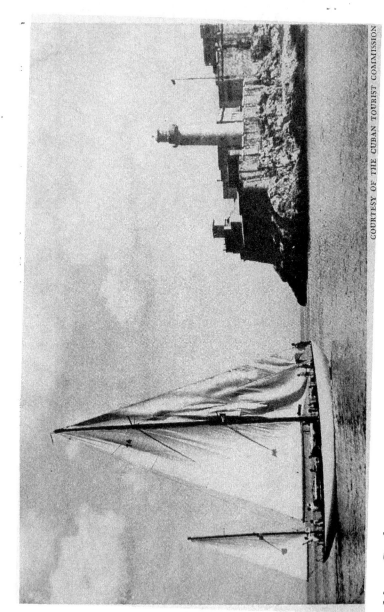

Morro Castle

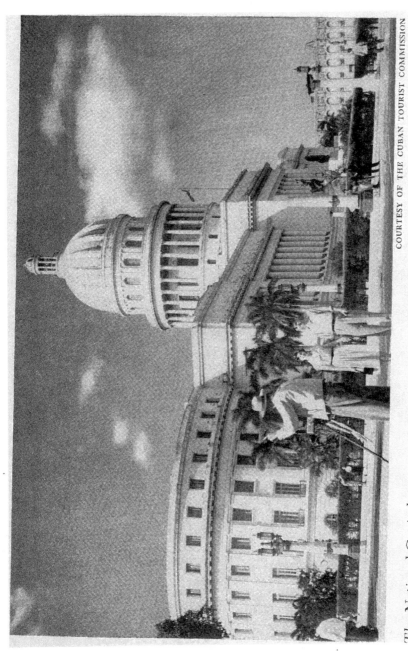

The National Capitol

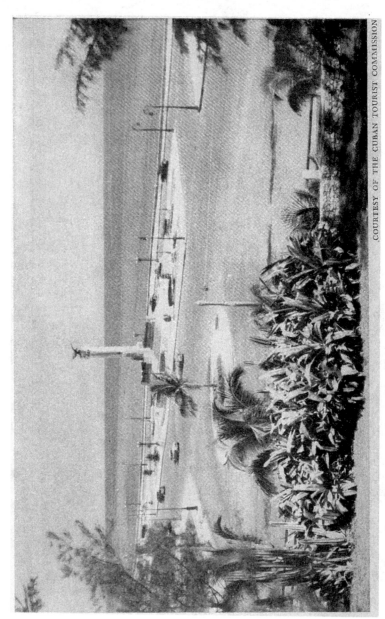

View of the Maine Plaza and Memorial

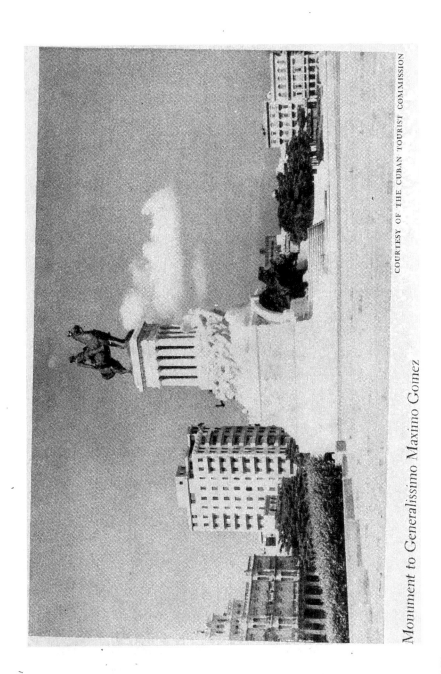

Monument to Generalissimo Maximo Gomez

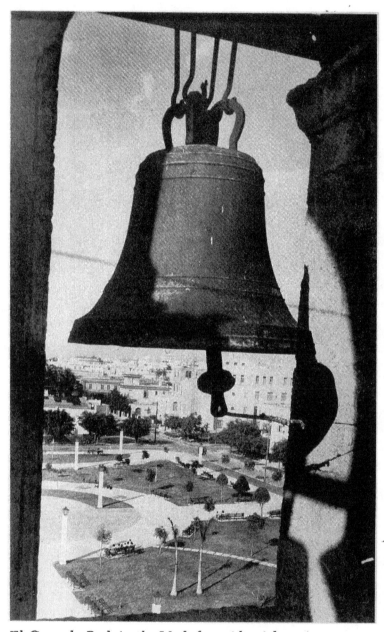

El Carmelo Park in the Vedado residential section

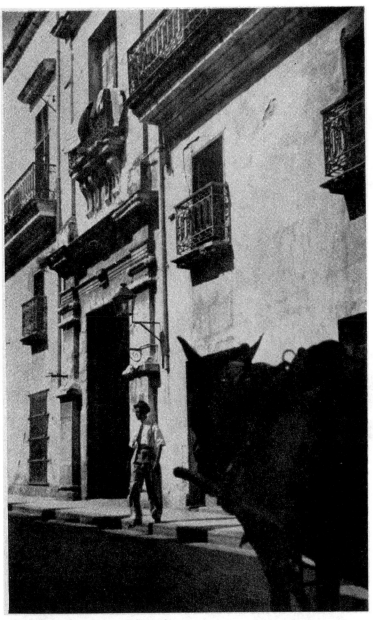

A colonial street in old Havana

Obispo Street

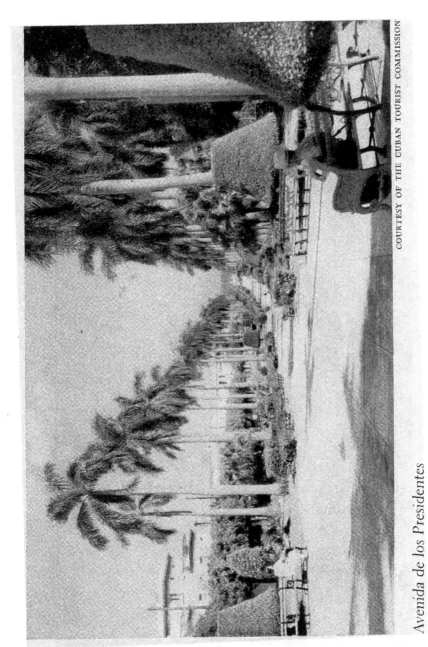

Avenida de los Presidentes

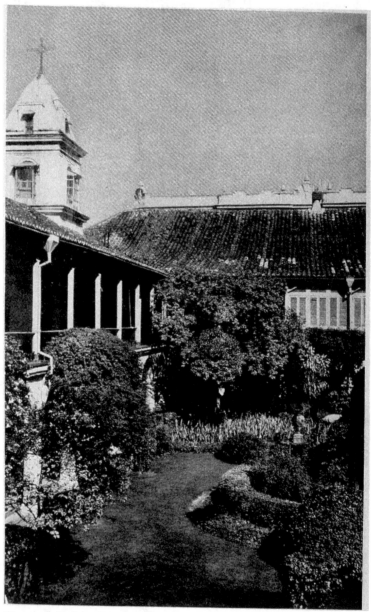

Typical Cuban Hacienda

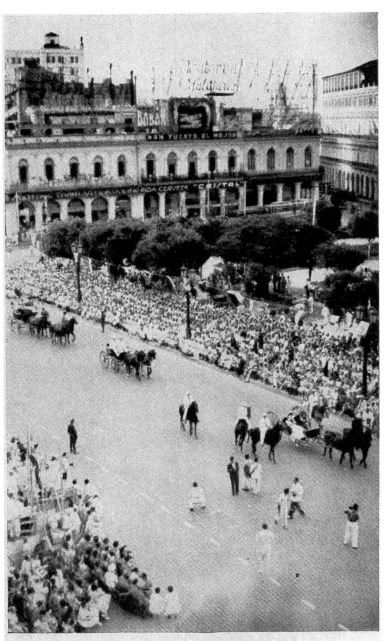

Parade through the streets of Havana

Jai-Alai

did not have it in him to be a popular leader. He was conservative and the suspicion grew that he did not intend to purge the army of the high officers who had supported Machado. An extraordinary movement then got under way. Led by the sergeant-stenographer Fulgencio Batista, the non-commissioned officers rose in revolt against their superiors, chased them into hiding, and took over the armed forces. Batista assumed the rank of colonel and at once became in effect the chief of staff. He was in his early thirties, a man of mixed blood including Chinese, the son of a truck gardener and quite unknown to the country. But his organizing talent soon made itself felt. He was to be the boss of Cuba for the next eleven years, part of the time openly. ·

Batista deposed Céspedes, who had been in office three weeks. He made the coup look better by asking the collaboration of the ABC and the students' committees, which also wanted to get rid of Céspedes. Dr. Grau, the anatomy professor, was given the office, and he showed sympathy for the ideas of militant youth rather than those of the more moderate ABC or the army. The term *auténticos* was used to describe the boy statesmen, who claimed to be the "authentics" of the revolution; it has persisted to this day as the name of a party, though the current membership can hardly be said to bear a strong resemblance to the 1933 founders. Eduardo Chibás was the archetype and he, at least, remained consistent to the end.

Grau had promised reforms, and he went about them radically by decree. A foreign-owned electric company was seized and its rates reduced by 45 per cent. Payment on Machado's largest American loan was stopped. Votes for women, the eight-hour day, a social-security system, workmen's compensation, and maternity insurance were put into effect. Batista found all this extreme. But it gratified the people, and for the moment he was busy recasting the military machine and liquidating the cashiered officers. Most of the latter, some four hundred of them, had congregated in the Nacional, a new American-owned hotel on the site of the Santa Clara Battery. It was and still is the largest, most luxurious hotel in Havana. Fate had decreed for it an immediate baptism as a historical building.

Batista ordered the officers to surrender. They elected to resist, though they had fewer than fifty rifles, a small store of revolvers, and very little ammunition. The place was then closely invested, its water and electric services cut off, its approaches commanded by fieldpieces and machine guns. It looked as if this would suffice to convince the officers, but they had a fair supply of food and they held out day after day without much shooting on either side. It was rumored that the besiegers had set October 2nd as the deadline. They said afterward that an officer fired the first shot that morning. The hotel was then bombarded, its main entrance smashed, balconies on the land side torn away, and the windows riddled with bullets. Batista personally directed the operations. Many of the officers were crack shots and they gave a good account of themselves, driving back several charges. When they surrendered at four in the afternoon for lack of cartridges, they had lost seventeen men while fifty-three of the attackers had been killed. The wounded on both sides exceeded two hundred.

It was now commonly supposed that Batista would make himself president. Nothing would have been easier, for the Battle of the Hotel Nacional had solidified his prestige. He chose to pull strings and exercise the real power. Grau was tolerated for four months, then ousted and driven into exile. The interlude of student domination ended simultaneously. The doctor and some of the lads would one day be back, but in a less idealistic mood.

Batista did a shrewd thing when he elevated Carlos Mendieta to the provisional presidency. It will be recalled that this noted Liberal and veteran of the War of Independence had been Machado's opponent for the nomination in 1924. Had he won, Cuba would have been spared great misery, and it seemed only right to give him his chance at last. Some of the politicians wondered how he could bring himself to take orders from a former sergeant-stenographer. The fact was that the two men worked together in a special way. Batista merely offered suggestions, and the rather solemn old Liberal was easily persuaded that he had originated them himself.

Mendieta had the approval of the United States. Franklin D. Roosevelt made him almost a personal beneficiary of the "Good Neighbor" policy by announcing in June, 1934, that the Platt Amendment had been abrogated. This completed Cuba's mastery of her own house, and coming so soon after the Machado terror it implied exceptional confidence in the new regime. The public gave Mendieta the credit, though this was more deserved by his brilliant secretary of state, Cosme de la Torriente. Mendieta enjoyed his two years in the palace, while Batista diligently constructed an ironbound political machine.

In 1936 it was decided to hold presidential elections. The choice of Batista fell on Miguel Mariano Gómez, ex-mayor of Havana and son of the popular second president whose memory was still green. There seemed no harm in putting forward as his running mate the oldish Federico Laredo Bru, a man of the War of Independence though with a dubious record in politics. The pair won easily. But Gómez became a sorry victim of the dictatorship. He tried, none too vigorously, to shape his own policies, and for this he was voted out of office seven months afterward by Congress in sheer violation of the constitution. Laredo Bru served out the term as the mouthpiece of Batista.

The last-named finally took the presidency in 1940, after an election in which he defeated Grau. There can be no doubt that between the collapse of Céspedes and the ejection of Gómez, Batista was a manipulator who usually had his way, and that after that he was a despot. Some of the evils of the Machado regime reappeared. The opposition was roughly treated. By comparison, however, it was a mild dictatorship and the opinion of the country was always taken into account. Batista had a sense of patriotism. His record was progressive in the fields of education, hygiene and public works. He had a certain *hombría* (maleness, though the precise Spanish connotation is untranslatable), which won him the liking of many who condemned his politics.

In September, 1941, ex-President Menocal died and was given a state funeral that surpassed in size that of José Miguel Gómez twenty years before. More than 200,000 persons followed Menocal's coffin to Colón Cemetery, where 5,000 other mourners had gathered.

As Batista's term drew to a close in 1944, he concluded that he would step behind the scenes once more. Apparently feeling sure that his faction could not be defeated, he backed Carlos Saladrigas for president and permitted an honest election. Dr. Grau ran again as the champion of the principles which had inspired the revolution against Machado and which had ever since been thwarted. There must have been a naive streak after all in the tough Batista, or he would never have been trustful that such dynamite could lose its detonating power in eleven years. Grau swept the country. Whispers of an armed coup to reverse the decision were heard. But Batista transferred the power peacefully, which counted then and afterward in his favor. He found it prudent to go into temporary exile, as had been the case with Grau in 1934.

His program unhampered even by threats, the new president had a wonderful chance to be the republic's best ruler. Unfortunately it did not turn out that way. Grau respected civil rights, and he forwarded the interests of labor by ending abuses, increasing wages, and shortening the hours of work. Morally he had lost stature since the early days. Always a bizarre personality, he had become morbid, gloomy. Little by little he surrounded himself with corrupt associates, and his administration was marked by colossal graft. Chibás and other idealists abandoned him. His hold on the people seriously declined.

Yet Grau was able to engineer the nomination and election of a member of his cabinet, Carlos Prio, to succeed him in 1948. The balloting was quiet and there was virtually no fraud. Batista, contesting *in absentia*, obtained a seat in the Senate. One of the candidates against Prio was Eduardo Chibás, who ran third. The comradeship between these two men in the Machado period ended with the minority zealot denouncing his fellow as a tool of the dishonored Grau.

Prio quickly showed, however, that he was not under the thumb of his predecessor. He broke with Grau in a few months, and although somewhat lacking in force and social vision his regime was superior to that of Grau. The chief trouble was that it, too, was shot through with graft. Prio made an affable, smiling president, who reveled in being liked personally and who found it hard to say *no* to his friends and relatives.

Toward the middle of the term, Chibás embarked upon a campaign of relentless criticism of all that Grau and Prio stood for, not to mention Batista. Members of the cabinet whom he had charged with gross irregularities threatened that he would be punished for libel, but he paid no heed. His dissident party, the *Ortodoxos*, nominated him far in advance for the presidency in the 1952 elections. Chibás, with his round boyish face and fanatical manner, created a mixed impression. No one doubted his sincerity; many thought him too neurotic to be a good chief of state, and he was easy to ridicule. Deciding that his message was not being taken seriously enough, he did an extraordinary thing to compel attention. He drew a revolver as he finished his scheduled speech over the air on August 5, 1951, and shot himself through the body.

The act of Chibás would have been dismissed in a phlegmatic northern country as that of a lunatic. It was emotionally understood in Cuba and had the effect of martyrdom. Chibás had not succeeded in killing himself outright. He succumbed nine days layer. Popular adulation of him had by then grown to gigantic proportions. His body was viewed by tens of thousands as it lay in the Aula Magna of the university. His funeral cortege was the largest Havana had ever known. Voluntary guards of honor stood at the tomb, day and night, for weeks. Professor Roberto Agramonte, of the University of Havana, was nominated by the Ortodoxos in place of Chibás and seemed to have the best chance of being elected president.

But on March 10, 1952, Fulgencio Batista overthrew the government in a *coup d'état* backed solidly by the army. He struck at three o'clock in the morning, and in a little longer than an hour he had control of Camp Columbia, the presidential palace, and all other important centers of power. The "Coup of Sunsundamba" was what the Negroes picturesquely called it, Sunsundamba being in Congo myth a night bird possessed by a spirit which if properly petitioned will help human beings.

Batista took the office of premier and appointed a cabinet. He then made every effort to legalize his course. He tried to get Prio and others in the line of succession to resign, so that he could be chosen president of the Senate. This would automatically have raised him to the acting presidency of the republic. The resignations were not forthcoming. Prio was allowed to go into exile in Mexico, and Batista suggested to the Congress that it declare the presidency vacant. When this was refused he informed Congress that it would not be allowed to sit during the rest of its term and that the general elections were postponed until November, 1953.

The next step was irregular. The cabinet adopted statutes amending the constitution, and by their authority appointed Batista to the provisional presidency. He in his turn nominated a body of eighty men and women, to be called the Consultative Council of the Nation and to exercise the functions of an advisory legislature. Legal or not legal, the good will shown by the dictator in setting up such a body made an excellent impression. That Batista immediately drove to cover the grafters and gangsters of the Prio regime is not to be denied. Havana became a safer, quieter city than it had been for years. Batista did not censor the press, but allowed all his moves to be criticized freely. Much has been written for and against him. But only the future can show whether he did well or ill to take arbitrary action in the very year that Cuba celebrated her first fifty years as an independent country.

PART II   **Havana Today**

Chapter 21

A ROVER'S VIEW

Most visitors in the old days saw Havana for the first time from the deck of a ship, with the Morro on the one side and the Punta on the other. Now the great majority come by plane and land at the Rancho Boyeros airport seventeen miles from the city. But whether they choose some outlying hotel or one at the center they soon realize that the Prado is the heart of things. It is the place from which to start out to note the sights, the restaurants, and the shops. I have always stayed on the Prado or within easiest reach of it. As I am the guide, let us rove in my preferred manner, afoot, and get impressions before I begin to classify the "musts."

Havana, at least for the tourist, is not an early-morning city. If you are up at eight o'clock, or a little before, the streets appear comparatively dead, except of course for employees hurrying to their jobs. The custom of sea-bathing on the downtown waterfront, which Dana described (see Chapter 14) no longer prevails. You are likely to have had breakfast at your hotel, at one of the restaurants run by Chinamen that serve American meals, or sitting at a circular counter Miami-style. If you want to do as the Cubans do, however, it can be interesting.

There are innumerable small cafés where the patrons order nothing but the good local beverage made by pouring a little essence of coffee into a cup of hot milk, and buttered toast, rusks, or biscuits. The best bread is called *pan flauta*. It is generally possible to get juice or sliced fruit at the café. But the Cuban takes his hot drink first, reads his newspaper and then moves on to a fruit counter, which may be a hole-in-the-wall or something quite elaborate. I have seen as many as twenty-three varieties of tropical fruits, nuts and the drinks derived from them listed above a counter. Pursued in this leisurely way, a Havana breakfast is cheap and also gives an insight into manners and customs.

The next stop should be the Prado, the most delightful of streets at any time of day. From the waterfront to the Parque Central its raised promenade of mottled, reddish marble is shadowed by a thick canopy of laurels. The sidewalks on the far sides of the two driveways are in part under arcades, and at every few steps you find novelty shops, refreshment places, theaters, clubs, and travel offices. This is the lower Prado. The Parque Central, of no great size, is flanked by imposing structures such as the Centro Gallego and the Centro Asturiano, which are the homes of mutual aid societies, and the Manzana de Gómez, a combined office building and shopping mart. Beyond this park the upper Prado runs in front of the Capitolio and merges with the Parque de la Fraternidad.

Dally in the lower Prado. There are marble benches with high backs and broad armrests on its promenade, which the sanitary department sluices with water at sunrise until they gleam. The sea looks wonderfully blue at the end of the tunnel formed by the laurels. On most mornings a fresh, light breeze rustles the foliage and starts to give way by nine o'clock to the languid balminess of the tropics. Types of all Havana dally along with you: solid citizens and ne'er-dowells, politicians deep in arguments, nursemaids with children, mysterious ancients, and girls of the demimonde who have not yet gone to bed. It is the traditional place for finishing the morning paper and having your shoes shined.

Shift now to the upper Prado. The Capitolio stands in fine grounds and is approached by an ample sweep of steps. The buildings opposite remain, with an insouciance not uncommon in Latin cities, a jumble from older days. It is true that at the western end the Teatro Payret has lately been rebuilt, while at about the middle the newspaper *El Diario de la Marina* is erecting an addition to its home. But the rest are hotels which have divided their once splendid lobbies into stores, some cheap rooming houses, shops of the kind that are always announcing sales, run-down motion picture theaters, photographers' studios, restaurants, and cafés. The last-mentioned improve the scene, for several of them have expanded onto the sidewalk and maintain the best open-air drinking places in Havana.

The entire frontage has its points, as a matter of fact. Nowhere else are there so many fruit-juice stands and tiny counters that sell coffee in cups of graded size, at two, three and five cents a cup. You readily fall into the Cuban habit of pausing often for a cooling glass, or a mouthful of stimulant which at that time of day is the better for not being alcoholic.

Back in the Parque Central you turn, if you have consulted your map, between the Manzana de Gómez and Centro Asturiano buildings. For this plunges you at once into Old Havana, by way of the Plazuela de Albear. Obispo and O'Reilly, the two oldest and narrowest shopping streets, extend before you to the harbor, the first to the right and the second to the left. They are crowded with traffic. The windows of dealers in cosmetics, jewelry, *objets d'art*, and books compete with the severe fronts of banks and the garish display of an American ten-cent store, while lottery-ticket agents spread their wares on the limited sidewalks. There are no awnings to meet above, as in days gone by, and the powerful tropical glare smites down upon the turmoil. But interest cannot flag. You drink another fruit juice, perhaps the water of a green coconut, and saunter on to the Plaza de Armas and the waterfront. Side forays into other ancient streets will suggest themselves, and my advice is to yield to any impulse. All of Old Havana is fascinating.

For luncheon I repeat the advice I have been in the habit of giving. Select some famous, high-priced place with its guarantee of elbow-room, or else a small one off the beaten track. The average downtown restaurant here could challenge a Times Square, New York, luncheon spot for congestion. After you have eaten it would be well to take a siesta. The Spaniards knew what they were about when they adopted that custom in hot countries.

In the afternoon it will be natural to rove the other side of the city, or New Havana. You are a pedestrian and will not be able to get very far into the huge quarter. It does not matter. You are only sampling. Neptuno, San Rafael and Galiano are shopping streets which carry forward the retail commerce they began in the last century (see Chapter 15). There are department stores large and small, as well as endless specialty shops. Many of the important cigar and cigarette manufactories are in this part of Havana. Chinatown occupies a large district west of Galiano and south of Zanja. Good restaurants are plentiful. You will find the two chief jai-alai *frontones* and numerous other amusement resorts.

If you are energetic you may stroll out to the Hotel Nacional and then return along the Malecón. I do not recommend all this walking for everyone, mind you. Most visitors will prefer to ride in taxis, and the public bus system covers the city with a network of more than thirty lines. But there is no beating the slow ramble if you are to absorb certain aspects of the spirit of a town. The Malecón, for example, is a marvel in the late afternoon, and the motorist who speeds along it will lose half of the effect. Though sea and sky may be suavely azure, there is usually enough of a breeze to toss spray above the embankment, and the west becomes a conflagration at sunset. On the land side noble monuments in a long succession break the regularity of tinted Mediterranean-style mansions and apartment houses.

So you wind up at the Prado once more. It is time for a cocktail, and the choice of bars is almost as wide as that of beverages. Absinthe, which is prohibited in most countries nowadays, can be had in Cuba. Plain vermouth, dubonnet, and various bitters are popular here as appetizers. The typical native cocktails are made with rum. Best known is undoubtedly the frozen *daiquirí*, called after the seacoast village near Santiago where United States troops first landed. The recipe is simple: pale rum, lime juice, sugar, and crushed ice, thoroughly shaken. Also well-liked is the *presidente*, concocted of dark rum and resembling a Manhattan. The *Cuba Libre*, invented to suit the North American taste, is a mixture of rum and Coca-Cola with a squeeze of lemon peel. But standard cocktails or *apéritifs* drunk anywhere in the world are perfectly familiar to the Havana bartenders.

Where to dine is a subject that will be discussed in a later chapter. Afterward, whether or not you go to a theater or night club, save the final hour for the lower Prado. The extraordinary character of the street is then more salient than at any other time. The benches are full and the marble promenade fairly effervesces with movement. Thousands share the same idea that occurred to you; they have come for a *paseo* before they go to bed—or in many cases to finish an argument. There is a rippling of laughter, a continuous babbling of voices. Overhead, birds rustle amidst the foliage of the laurels, for oddly enough, great flocks of black grackles which feed in the country return at dusk to roost on the branches above the street that is most frequented by human beings.

I have shown that I consider it a charming city. But nothing is perfect. There is one feature about Havana which I detest, and that is the preposterous, incessant blowing of horns by motorists. I am told that when the automobile first came into general use about forty-five years ago it was held, with some justice, to be a dangerous contraption and chauffeurs were ordered by law to sound a warning at every street crossing. The habit then acquired has become a mania, and in the event of a traffic jam the drivers show their wrath or hilarity by blasting away at one another. It is also said that Cubans like to show off their possession of a car by leaning on the klaxon. Anyway, the custom is senseless. Other cities have found that when horn-blowing is forbidden except in serious warning, the number of accidents decreases. It would be an aid to tourism if the national and municipal administrations would take action to abolish this nuisance. A survey made early in 1952 established that 85.38 per cent of the unnecessary noise in Havana was caused by automobiles, motor cycles, and buses.

After all, the population of Havana proper is in round figures 725,000, while the total urban center has more than 800,000 inhabitants. It is too large a community to continue to tolerate childish practices where noise is concerned.

Chapter 22

STREET NAMES OF HAVANA

AN IDIOSYNCRASY of the Havana public is to refuse
to accept the renaming of prominent streets. The city fathers, on the other hand, have tried to honor national
heroes and compliment foreign countries by christening old
thoroughfares afresh. They have passed ordinances, changed
the street signs and altered the maps. It is no go. The citizens continue to address mail and give directions according
to the ancient style. A taxi driver will throw you a puzzled
glance if you mention an appellation that has been staring
him in the face for years, and at last will mutter, "Oh, you
mean so-and-so!" This is hard on visitors who have not had
time to work out the riddle by a trial and error system.
Charts with double indications have had to be printed.

It adds piquancy to the whole subject, of course. I have
been using the traditional names in these pages. Now let us
review the more interesting examples.

El Prado. This is the common word in Spanish for a public walk; it also means a field. It was being used when Tacón
renovated the promenade outside the walls of Havana about
a century and a quarter ago and decreed the name Paseo de
Isabel II. The populace went on saying Prado. The republic
officially changed it to the Paseo de Martí, and although
there is no more venerated figure in Cuban history than
Martí, it remains the Prado in everyday parlance.

Calle Obispo. The word *obispo* means bishop. An early prelate had his house at the corner of the Plaza de Armas and this street, hence the name. The republic called it Pi y Margall after a Spanish historian who had spoken up for Cuba, and there never was so dead a letter as that one.

Calle O'Reilly. Named in honor of General Alexander O'Reilly, the Irish "wild goose" who commanded the Spanish forces that took over Havana when it was evacuated by the English in 1763. O'Reilly later pacified New Orleans, which had been ceded against its will to Spain. Determined efforts have been made to alter the name to Presidente Zayas. The new signs are in place from end to end of the street. Except for a few provincials and foreigners, O'Reilly is what people use. The Havanese do not care much, anyhow, for the memory of the fourth president, Alfredo Zayas.

Calle Empedrado. Meaning paved. It runs in front of the cathedral and was the first paved street in Havana, cobblestones being used. Beyond the cathedral plaza it is extremely narrow. General Riva's name is now attached to it, uselessly.

Calle Paula. Took its name from the hospital of San Francisco de Paula that stood at the end of it. Renamed Leonor Pérez in honor of the mother of Martí, who gave birth to the great patriot in a house on this street which is now maintained as a national shrine and museum. Yet Paula clings.

Calle Amargura. The word means bitterness or sorrow. Early in the city's history, the Franciscans held religious processions on this street leading to a calvary on the spot where the Cristo church was later built. The route was venerated as a *Via Crucis.* The authorities made a futile gesture when they renamed it Marta Abreu for a distinguished Cuban woman.

Calle Teniente Rey. Called after a military auditor in

Spanish times, one Rey, who had his house on the street. However, *rey* means king, and Teniente Rey sounded romantic because it appeared to refer to some famous "lieutenant of the King." Its present official appellation of Brazil is ignored.

Avenida Monserrate. Named for a hermitage which once stood on part of the site of the Manzana de Gómez building. The attempt to please Belgium by giving that country's name to the avenue is a total failure. Monserrate used to run just outside the walls, in which there was a Puerta del Monserrate.

Calle Zulueta. Called after an old worthy. Renamed Ignacio Agramonte after one of the principal heroes of the Ten Years' War. But Zulueta hangs on.

Calle Bernaza. The seventeenth-century proprietor of a bakery left his name attached to this street. Now it is officially Plácido, after the mulatto poet who was executed in 1844 (see Chapter 13).

Calle Tacón. A street one block in length, running west from the south side of the Plaza de Armas. Changed to Roosevelt, after the Rough Rider, a name sometimes used because the memory of Captain General Tacón is not treasured in Havana.

Calle del Cárcel. Derives from the prison, long since demolished, alongside which it ran. Rechristened Capdevila for the Spanish captain who stoutly defended the martyred medical students in 1871—another change that is mildly favored.

Avenida del Puerto. The waterfront street within the harbor. Recently widened, greatly improved and called Céspedes, in honor of Carlos Manuel de Céspedes. He launched the Ten Years' War and was the first provisional president of Cuba. People still say Puerto, but are likely to adopt the new name because the avenue has taken on a new character.

Calle Neptuno. The streets mentioned up to this point are east of the Prado. We move westward. Neptuno, the god of the sea, was a logical name in maritime Havana. The public would not accept a change to Juan Clemente Zenea, after the beloved poet who was shot in the Cabaña fortress during the Ten Years' War.

Calle San Rafael. After a saint. The official name General Carrillo, bestowed under the republic, fell flat. The same is true of *San Miguel*, altered to General Suárez; and *San José*, altered to José de San Martín, the father of Argentine independence.

Calzada de la Reina. Called for some queen of Spain, probably Isabel II since it is in New Havana. The change to Avenida de Simón Bolívar is pretty generally ignored, despite popular admiration of the Liberator.

Calle del Monte. A commonplace name, for *monte* is broadly used to indicate a mountain, a forest, or just the bush. The street led toward wild country. Now it is officially Máximo Gómez, and as in the case of the Paseo de Martí one cannot help being surprised that the assignment to a great national hero should have failed of acceptance.

El Malecón. Another case like the above. Formally renamed Avenida de Antonio Maceo, it is the Malecón ("embankment, levee") to rich and poor in Havana.

Calle Virtudes. Meaning the "Virtues," after a masonic lodge of that name which was located in it. Assuredly it is no center of virtue today. The republic sought to rechristen it Major Gorgas in honor of the American officer who cleaned up Havana after the cause of yellow fever epidemics had been discovered, a worthy intention which simply no one will recognize.

Avenida de la Zanja. This is as ironical a case as the preceding one. *Zanja* means "ditch." Water used to be conveyed along this route from the Almendares River to the

city, by means of a ditch of doubtful salubrity where mosquitoes bred. Dr. Carlos Finlay, who made possible the conquest of yellow fever by advancing the mosquito theory
seemed the logical godfather. But will any one call it the
Avenida Finlay? No. It remains the street of the ditch.

Calle Consulado. A consulate, or a tribunal of commerce.
- The origin of the name is obscure. Changed ineffectively to
Estrada Palma, after the first President of Cuba.

Calle Amistad. Means "friendship." Altered to Aldama,
after the millionaire patriot of the Ten Years' War, whose
family mansion faces it. Amistad is tenaciously preferred.

Avenida San Lázaro. Saint Lazarus is often a patron of
hospitals and cemeteries. Both once stood on this avenue.
The new name of Republica is simply a designation on the
maps.

Paseo de Carlos III. Laid out by Captain General Tacón
(see Chapter 12), and popularly nicknamed for him then
and afterward. Carlos III holds firm, and no one pays any
attention to the official label of Independencia.

Avenida Galiano. An engineer who was in charge of
building fortifications gave his name to this important shopping thoroughfare. Now it is Italia, but never in popular
speech. The citizens do not merely say that such-and-such
a building is on Galiano. They refer to nearby streets as
being so many blocks this side, or that side of Galiano.

Calzada de la Infanta. The word means any daughter of
a king of Spain. Probably called after the Infanta Maria
Teresa, who gave her name also to the flagship of Admiral
Cervera which was sunk in the battle off Santiago de Cuba.
The avenue has become Presidente Menocal, with com-
mon acceptance for the future, if ever.

Calle de los Perros. Meaning the street of the dogs. Here
is a rare example of a change having been approved. The
street is only three blocks long and has been notorious for

its low houses of prostitution standing side by side. Perhaps a salacious jest was seen in the implication of female dogs. The public, at all events, now willingly says Calle Bernal.

Calle G. The streets and avenues in the Vedado are prosaically designated by numbers and the letters of the alphabet. This is not in the tradition of Latin countries, and the present tendency to rename them will probably be accepted in time. G has been changed to Avenida de los Presidentes, and Fifth to Avenida de las Americas. Old pre-suburban designations have been popularly revived for Seventh and Ninth; Calzada, or "paved highway," for the former; and Linea, or "boundary," for the latter.

Chapter 23

THE CATHEDRAL AND CHURCHES

As MIGHT BE EXPECTED in a city where there was no great devotion to the Church during the age of piety, Havana's ecclesiastical buildings are not of the first order of merit. Some of course are interesting architecturally, some dowered with precious objects. But they have never housed celebrated works of art in the way of paintings and sculpture. The interiors are comparatively small, except for one or two that were erected in modern times. A liberal Cuban told me that, as he saw it, the earliest citizens were heedless, and those of the middle period associated the clergy with Spanish oppression, whereas under the republic, the Church had become fashionable. This would appear a sound explanation.

It is worth noting that the country never had a cardinal before Pope Pius XII gave the red hat in 1946 to Emanuel Arteaga y Betancourt, the archbishop of Cuba.

La Catedral has been mentioned previously (see Chapters 6, 8, and 9). It is on Empedrado at the corner of San Ignacio, and it faces a lovely old-world plaza named after it. The original church on this site was built by the Jesuits in 1674, and completely reconstructed between 1704 and 1724. When the Order was expelled from the Spanish dominions in 1767, the structure was taken over by the regular Church authorities and in 1789 it was made the cathedral of the diocese of Havana. Often called the Colón (Columbus) Cathedral for reasons which will appear below, or San Cristóbal because of a mistaken idea that it was dedicated in honor of the Discoverer, its real name is La Virgen Maria de la Concepción, or in English "the Virgin Mary of the Immaculate Conception."

The edifice, which has two irregular towers and a shallow dome, is a mixture of Spanish baroque and what is known in Spain as Jesuit. Hence the numerous columns and the many niches. The style of the façade in churches of the sort throughout colonial America may have been inspired by the temple of the cave of Manressa, where Ignatius Loyola, the founder of the Society of Jesus, did penance. This cathedral is built of the native limestone, which is yellowish-white when quarried; but the surface soon darkens and crumbles, giving the appearance of great age.

Inside, the colored marbles, greenish glass and light-tinted walls create an astonishing effect of brightness. A shadowy interior would be more impressive. The main altar of Carrara marble gleams with gold, silver, onyx, and carved woods. A little of the sculpture is of historical interest. The niche in the left wall of the chancel where the casket containing the supposed bones of Christopher Columbus (see Chapter 9) was placed in 1796 is appropriately marked. But it is empty. The Spaniards took the relics with them when they evacuated Havana on January 1, 1899.

Through a passage to the right you may enter the ecclesiastical reception room, the walls of which are hung with portraits of dead bishops. The cloisters and the patio of the Theological Seminary of San Carlos lie beyond. In the patio, on the exterior wall of the cathedral, is a tablet to Pierre le Moyne, Sieur d'Iberville, the founder of Louisiana, who died of yellow fever on his ship in Havana harbor in 1706 and was buried in the now demolished parish church (see Chapter 6). American, Canadian, and French residents join every year in placing a floral wreath below the Iberville memorial.

The treasure room of the cathedral may be visited for a small fee. It contains antique vestments heavy with gold embroidery, a celebrated monstrance of solid silver weighing six hundred pounds, plate, jewelry, and paintings.

Colonial palaces, which have been restored, stand on three sides of the small plaza and furnish an admirable setting for the cathedral. On bright moonlight nights when traffic has been reduced to a minimum, the whole effect is magical. Nowhere else in Havana does the atmosphere of bygone centuries linger so subtly.

El Templete, at the northeastern edge of the Plaza de Armas (see Chapter 2), is a chapel dedicated to Christopher Columbus in the year 1828. One of the three paintings on its walls commemorates the legend that the spot was the scene of the first mass said in Havana. The other two portray a municipal council in Santiago presided over by Velásquez, the first governor of Cuba; and the inauguration of

El Templete itself. There is a good bust of Columbus in the front court, and the column standing there marks the site of the original ceiba tree.

Dr. Roig de Leuchsenring considers the cathedral the finest church in Havana. He gives second place to the old church and convent of San Francisco now occupied by the General Post Office, and says that all the other churches—interiors as well as exteriors—are lacking in architectural artistic values.

Old *San Francisco* (see Chapters 4 and 7), as reconstructed in the early eighteenth century, is a bulky and somber period-piece which appears to be almost as much a fortress as a church. This impression is enhanced by its location on the waterfront. The tower, which has three floors, was in fact used as a lookout for approaching ships. It contains statuary honoring Saints Francis and Dominic, founders of the religious orders bearing their names. Eleven cells of the ancient monastery front the patio, beneath the pavement of which many of the monks lie buried. When the Department of Communications gives up the building, it will probably be used as a museum.

New *San Francisco*, belonging to the Order of St. Francis of Assisi, is situated on Cuba near Amargura. It was entirely reconstructed on ancient foundations in 1925. Formerly Augustinian monks had a convent there.

Santa Clara Convent. Like the old San Francisco church, this convent is in use by the government. It houses the Department of Public Works. Completed about 1635 (see Chapters 2 and 6) and only slightly modified since, it remains an excellent example of the oldest type of good building done in Havana. The patio is especially interesting, for three antique structures have been preserved there: a slaughter house of midget proportions, a fountain with baths, and the so-called "fisherman's house" which is said

to have been built by a seafaring man for his daughter. No
visitor should miss this patio. A cemetery containing the
bodies of nuns may be seen, a few steps from the long
ranges of cells which they occupied in life.

Cristo church on Cristo Plaza, Villegas and Amargura,
was built in the middle of the seventeenth century, and it
too represents the earliest Spanish architecture in Havana.
Its two towers rise above a unique tiled roof. Augustinian
fathers conduct many of the services in English for the
benefit of travelers and resident English-speaking Catholics.
The interior is plain, but harmonious.

Angel church, the full name of which is La Iglesia del
Santo Angel Custodia, also dates from the seventeenth century. The Jesuit Order founded it in 1672. The style is
Gothic, but with a decidedly over-decorated, or baroque,
interior. It was once an auxiliary of the cathedral, when the
parent edifice was Jesuit. There are ten chapels, the most
important of them being that of the Holy Sacrament, situated behind the high altar. The medallions in the ceiling
are the work of the Catalan painter Manuel Roig. The
church stands on a hill named La Loma de Peña Pobre,
often referred to as La Loma del Angel. The action of the
classic Cuban novel, *Cecilia Valdés*, by Cirilo Villaverde
(see Chapter 10) is set in the Angel quarter, and one of its
tragic scenes takes place on the steps of the church. Appropriately, a bust of Villaverde has been erected opposite the
main entrance.

Paula church is a small eighteenth-century building on
the waterfront at the foot of the Calle Paula. It has charm.
No longer in use, it was spared as a historic monument
when the Avenida del Puerto was widened and improved.

La Merced. This church, at Cuba and Merced, though
located at the somewhat run-down eastern end of Old
Havana, is the richest and most fashionable in the city. It

was erected in 1746, reconstructed in 1792, and the interior remodeled and decorated with great splendor in recent years. It has many fine chapels. The altars are of marble. The lavish paintings are chiefly memorable for their associations with Cuban history. A valuable treasure in plate, jewelry and vestments has been accumulated.

El Sagrado Corazón. This large new church with a tall spire, on Reina at Belascoain, is modeled after the Gothic cathedral in León, Spain. It was completed in 1923. The stained glass windows were made in France at a cost of $54,000. The high altar is of Spanish make and cost $72,-000. Sagrado Corazón almost equals Merced in wealth.

Carmen church, on Infanta and Compostela, is another huge and comparatively modern structure. It has little to recommend it from the artistic point of view.

Monserrate church, Galiano and Concordia, was built in the last century to replace the Monserrate hermitage that disappeared when the city walls were torn down. The present building succeeds in being both gaudy and commonplace.

Until the Spaniards were driven from Cuba in 1898, Protestant sects were not allowed to worship in public. The bishop of Havana even rejected a plea that the Episcopalian burial service be read at the funeral of the Protestants who had died in the explosion of the armored cruiser *Maine*. Today the Episcopalians have a cathedral, *Holy Trinity*, which used to stand at Neptuno and Aguila, and is now completed at 13th and 6th in the Vedado. The Methodists have a large church at the corner of Virtudes and Industria, while other denominations are represented. Complete freedom of worship prevails in the Republic of Cuba.

Chapter 24

THE CAPITOL AND THE PALACE

THE CAPITOL (El Capitolio) is without rivalry the most imposing modern building in Havana, though I could wish that Cuba had had enough originality to adopt some other form of architecture than the Graeco-Roman of the United States Capitol, which the exterior closely resembles. It faces the upper Prado just beyond the Parque Central and stands in its own grounds. The site used to be occupied by the Villanueva railroad station of the Ferrocarriles Unidos de la Habana, which itself had caused the destruction of an old botanical garden. The Villanueva station had been a center of conspiracy in all Cuba's struggles for freedom. Most of the railroad employees were secret revolutionaries, and through them it was practicable to communicate with the leaders in the interior.

A capitol was planned as early as the administration of José Miguel Gómez, the second president. The Villanueva lands were then acquired by the government, the idea being to erect there a presidential palace, office buildings for various departments, and a comparatively small capitol. The last-mentioned was started, but the work languished because the immediate successors of Gómez thought the project inadequate. Under Zayas (1921-25) the unfinished capitol was abandoned, and when Machado succeeded him as president it was demolished to make place for the present great structure built on the entire Villanueva site. It was one of Machado's pet schemes for earning credit for his regime (see Chapter 19) and he pushed the work through in time to dedicate the Capitol on May 20, 1929.

A little smaller than the United States Capitol, but relatively much larger when one considers the sizes of the two countries, as Cubans like to say, this capitol is ahead in certain respects. It has a higher dome, a larger reception hall, an indoor statue far taller than any in Washington. The dome ranks third in the whole world, the highest being that of St. Peter's in Rome, and the second that of St. Paul's in London.

The great Cuban salon is 400 feet long, 45 feet wide, and 65 feet high: against the wall at its center stands the statue of the Republic by the Italian sculptor Angelo Zanelli, 58 feet tall including its base and exceeded indoors only by a figure of Buddha in Japan. Kilometer zero of Cuba's road system is marked by a diamond embedded in the floor at the foot of the statue. This gem is valued at between $30,000 and $40,000. It was pried out and stolen about seven years ago in circumstances so inexplicable that cynics at once declared it must have been "an inside job." A few months later it was anonymously returned by ordinary parcel post from Miami, Florida.

The reception hall is known as the Salón de los Pasos Perdidios, or "Hall of Lost Footsteps." The President takes the oath of office there, and it is the scene of receptions on national holidays. Beautiful marbles and immense bronze chandeliers adorn it. Scarcely less sumptuous, though smaller, is the Martí Salon which of course features a bust of the Apostle, a very large one. Its paintings and decorations are Pompeiian in style. State banquets are given there. It serves as a lobby to the congressional library on

international law and relations, which contains more than
50,000 volumes. The library and the various conference
rooms are provided with mahogany furniture of admirable
design.

As in Washington, the Senate and the House of Representatives sit at opposite ends of the building. In the first
chamber, the original flag of the single star carried by
Narciso López in 1850 is framed upon the wall beside
the chair of the presiding officer. The House displays in
similar fashion the banner raised by Carlos Manuel de
Céspedes in 1868, and there is also an elaborate high-relief
illustrating Peace and War.

Statuary and paintings of presidents, legislators, and soldiers abound. I wish I could say that most of them have
artistic merit. A huge double panel in bronze arrests the
attention. It portrays episodes from the history of Cuba.
The last section glorified Machado himself, but it was
ripped out with a crowbar after the fall of the despot in
1933.

At ground level at the center of the building is the
entrance to a shrine which tourists almost never visit.
Guides, for some reason, do not call attention to it. This
is the crypt of the Tomb of the Unknown Mambí Soldier.
(It will be recalled that a Mambí was a patriot in arms
against Spain.) The sarcophagus is surrounded by six
bronze figures which represent the six provinces of Cuba.

Generally speaking, the impression made by the Capitol
is one of overwhelming luxury. It need not have been anything so large or ornate for practical purposes. So it must
be judged as a monument, and as such it is splendid, an
assertion of pride in national independence. Cubans brush
aside the memory of Machado in connection with it.

The Presidential Palace, between Monserrate and Zulueta, close to the waterfront and looking down the land-

scaped Avenida Missiones, is a building which has been criticized because it is a mixture of several styles of architecture. The irreverent have even said that with its florid exterior details and dome it resembles a wedding cake. I cannot agree that it is unattractive. The spirit of southern Spain has been captured, oddly influenced by the Renaissance. At all events, it is more original than the neo-classic Capitol. The most astonishing thing about the Palace is the almost purely French atmosphere that prevails inside. It is furnished and decorated like a little Versailles.

General Menocal was the first President to live there. His personal taste had a great deal to do with the style, or combination of styles, adopted. The building had been started to house the administrative departments of the Province of Havana. Menocal liked it, and as the plan for a palace on the Villanueva lands had fallen through he influenced Congress to acquire the half-finished structure on Missiones. Thereafter he supervised the changes made.

The Palace consists of a ground floor at street level and three upper stories. On the ground floor are the quarters of the military guard and various service installations. There are elevators, of course, but you get a better visual effect by climbing the marble stairway. As soon as you reach the first story you are in a regal French château, modified only by the native scenes of the paintings on the walls and by certain pieces of fine old Creole mahogany furniture.

The paintings deserve attention. In the reception hall are a panel by Augusto Menocal showing the landing of Christopher Columbus in Cuba, another by Hurtado Mendoza of the burning at the stake of the heroic Indian cacique Hatuey, a third by Hernández Giró of a conference held by Martí, Gómez, and Maceo at the start of the War of Independence; and a fourth by Esteban Valderrama showing Dr. Carlos Finlay expounding his mosquito theory to the military commission headed by Major Walter Reed. These pictures are not of equal merit. Valderrama is, in my opinion, the most effective artist, and Hernández Giró the next best. But all the panels are of historical interest. At the far end of the room where the cabinet meets is another mural by Hernández Giró, portraying the convention at Guaimaro presided over by Carlos Manuel de Céspedes in the Ten Years' War. The ceilings of the ballroom and of a lesser salon are covered with vast allegorical paintings in the eighteenth-century Gallic manner.

Inevitable busts of heroes occur at every turn. Those featured in the reception hall are of Martí, Bolívar, Lincoln, and Benito Juarez of Mexico. Martí figures again in an admirable bust behind and above the chair where the President of Cuba sits to conduct the affairs of state. Ordinarily visitors are not shown this private office. But I was taken into it. It is furnished with great splendor. The chairs and lounges are of a pattern used by Napoleon. Martí's republic and the First Empire! The juxtaposition is beguiling.

A chapel in the palace contains an altar before which the Spanish captains general once worshipped. The top floor is given over to the living quarters of the president's family. One hears talk that this has been for some years regarded as a very exposed position. Buildings taller than the Palace stand close to it on two sides, and in a revolution snipers could rake it with rifle fire. The guns of the Cabaña Castle across the harbor could easily pound it into rubble. Therefore, it is said that a new palace may be erected in a park of its own on heights near the city, in which case the present one would be turned over to the Department of State.

The Presidential Palace may be visited if a permit has first been obtained through official channels.

Chapter 25
OTHER NOTABLE BUILDINGS

MUCH HAS BEEN SAID in the historical section of this book about the Municipal Palace, formerly the palace of the captains general of Cuba. It is the finest public building from the colonial period, and probably it should be regarded as more distinguished architecturally than either the new Capitol or the Presidential Palace. While not unique, it is a good example of late eighteenth-century Spanish. The original architect was Pedro de Medina, who completed it in 1790 as a residence, administrative headquarters, and jail. Tacón improved it in 1835 and shifted the prisoners to other quarters. Miguel Mariano Gómez, while mayor, had the entire structure restored in 1930.

The great reception salon is notably impressive, the patio with its palm trees and its statue of Columbus a lovely spot. The walls are of masonry, thick and strengthened by granite socles. Atop, with low battlements like those of a castle, the flat roof makes a quadrilateral walk around the patio. The main entrance is ornamented with two marble Corinthian columns set close against the wall, and the cornice above the portico is circular.

Generals Brooke and Wood occupied the palace as military governors during the American intervention. So did the first three presidents of the republic up till 1920. It was then turned over to the city of Havana.

171

To the left, facing the Plaza de Armas and behind La Fuerza, is the former palace of the Segundo Cabo ("second chief," or lieutenant governor), which also housed the post office and other administrative departments in Spanish days. It was completed in 1772 and is considered a solid and rather elegant variation of Spanish baroque. Under the republic it was the first home of the Cuban Senate, and after the latter moved to the Capitol in 1929 it became the seat of the Supreme Court. There is an interesting bust of Martí by Juan José Sicre in the patio.

The Aldama palace, Amistad and Reina (see Chapter 14), has been praised by architects in the highest terms as an example of majestic and harmonious beauty. It actually consisted of two dwellings so linked about a patio that they seemed one. The top story was added after the building had been looted during the Ten Years' War and had degenerated into commercial uses; it is a violation of taste, and the visitor should try to imagine that it is not there. Much damage was done when the structure was turned into a tobacco factory. But although it is now subdivided into stores and offices, there is recognition of the fact that it is an artistic heritage. The patio, the vast stairways and the decorative stonework have been in part restored. Had independence been won in his time, Miguel de Aldama intended to offer the palace as the residence of the chief executives of Cuba.

The four ancient palaces about the Plaza de la Catedral, along with the cathedral itself, compose a well-conceived restoration of colonial atmosphere. All of these mansions are meritorious. The one on the east side of the square, facing the cathedral, is the most obviously attractive, its patio thick with decorative palms and shrubs, its high-ceilinged rooms revealing lovely workmanship in stone and hardwoods. It was once the home of the Counts of Casa

Bayona, and is now in the possession of the Havana Rum Company, which deserves credit for keeping it in a good state of preservation. Any visitor who cares to drop in is entertained there.

As mentioned in the chapter on museums and libraries, the building on the northwest corner of the plaza is occupied by the Museum of the City of Havana. It used to be the palace of the Lombillo family, and architecturally it is of the same period and much the same standard as that of the Counts of Bayona. Its existence has often been threatened by commercial interests, but we may assume that the role now assigned to it makes it safe for posterity. Alongside it is the mansion of the Marquisses of Arcos, given over today to the manufacture and sale of goods in alligator leather.

On the south side the mansion occupied by the Restaurant Paris is called the palace of Ponce de León. The original conquistador who bore that name could have had nothing to do with it, for when he died in Havana after the failure of his quest for the Fountain of Youth in Florida the town consisted of thatch-roofed huts. Properly the mansion should be named for the Marquisses of Aguas Claras, who inherited it shortly after it was built.

The Centro Gallego and the Centro Asturiano cannot be omitted from any survey of Havana's fine buildings. They are the homes of great mutual-aid societies founded by immigrants from two of Spain's northern provinces, Galicia and Asturias, but now of unrestricted membership. Better sites could not have been obtained, for the Centro Gallego is on the Prado, beside the Capitol, and facing the Parque Central; while the Centro Asturiano is directly across the park. Their windows command a grandstand view of patriotic and carnival parades. The structures are magnificent, no less, in the manner of half a century ago when they were erected. You mount flights of marble stairs to vast salons where dances and receptions are held. The luxurious ornaments, exterior and interior, are exceeded only by those of the Capitol and the National Palace. Incorporated in the Centro Gallego and much modified is the Tacón Theater, now called the National Theater (Teatro Nacional).

The Casa de Beneficencia, facing the Parque Maceo, consists of a group of interesting convent buildings, some of them two hundred years old. The Casa is a home for orphans, founded in 1794 by Bishop Valdés. Anyone may leave a baby there by placing it on a shelf that is revealed when a small, low door on Belascoain is opened. The child is christened and given the family name of Valdés, but in some cases may be reclaimed by its parents. As it grows up it is taught a trade. The Casa de Beneficencia is in part supported by the National Lottery. It also enjoys several rich endowments bestowed upon it through the years.

Considered as a utilitarian office building that nevertheless has a pleasing appearance, the Manzana de Gómez on the Parque Central is worth mentioning. *Manzana* in this sense signifies a city block; it is also Spanish for an apple. Some of the banks have dignity, though they are conventional in their use of Graeco-Roman. It was poor taste to crowd the fluted columns of Cuba's national bank and treasury on Obispo, of all thoroughfares the one that could least furnish the needed visual approach.

The building of the Bacardí Rum Company, on Monserrate, is eccentric-looking, being flamboyant in the style of the 1920's. Vivid colors have been employed, and it is one of the few structures in Havana tall enough to qualify as a skyscraper.

Chapter 26
MUSEUMS AND LIBRARIES

THE NATIONAL MUSEUM has been housed for a number of years in a colonial mansion on Aguiar, between Amargura and Teniente Rey, but will be removed to a much more adequate building, a reconstruction of the old Colón Market behind the Presidential Palace. This work is now under way.

Interest is divided between the fine arts and relics of historical value in the museum. Most of the older canvases were salvaged from churches about to be pulled down or secularized, and except for a portrayal by José Ribera of an early Christian martyrdom it is doubtful if there are any original masterpieces among them. Copies abound. In other cases the work of imitators is to be earnestly suspected. The two Murillos, *Saint Isabel of Hungary* and *Madonna and Child*, are merely "attributed" to him. The same is true of the *Virgin and Child* of Guido Reni and the *Apollo and Mars* of Coreggio. Velázquez, Raphael, Rubens, Titian, and Veronese are represented by manifest copies. Watteau's *A Day in the Country* and Thomas Lawrence's *Portrait* are originals, but ordinary.

Of consequence to students of Cuban painting are the exhibits in the salon devoted to early native artists. José Nicolás de la Escalera (1734-1804) was the first whose work

175

has come down to us. Nearly all his subjects are religious, as for example his *St. Alipio, St. Anthony,* and *St. Joseph with the Child Jesus.* Vicente Escobar (1757-1854), who was of mixed blood, enjoyed a reputation as a portraitist; his *Christ Praying* and *Portrait of a Woman* are shown. Also see Miguel Angel Melero's *Battle of Champigni,* Juan Peoli's *Sculpture and Painting,* José Arburo's *The Man with the Sword,* Francisco Cisneros' *Lot and His Daughters,* and Ferrán's *Christ and the Woman of Samaria.*

Superior intrinsically are the canvases in the hall of contemporary painters, Spanish and Cuban. The great Ignacio Zuloaga has three, of which *My Cousin Esperanza* and *Woman with Fan* are particularly striking. Joaquin Sorolla has *Boy with Watermelon.* Leopoldo Romañach, *doyen* of the present generation of Cuban masters, who died in 1951, is represented.

The historical section of the National Museum cannot be said to be well organized, but this is largely due to the cramped space available. A museum in the outdated sense of being a repository for curios is just what it has been. You browse from room to room and come upon surprising things, such as the skeleton of the favorite war horse of the generalissimo Máximo Gómez, and the rowboat in which Antonio Maceo crossed the bay of Mariel during the War of Independence. There are souvenirs of Carlos Manuel de Céspedes, Jose Martí, and lesser heroes. Those in the arts are not overlooked. The women of Cuba receive much space. Weapons and costumes of every period are featured. The Latin penchant for the macabre is evident in such items as a photograph of Maceo's skull, made when his bones were disinterred from their temporary grave near the battlefield, and in many death masks of other national figures.

Artifacts of aboriginal life before the coming of Columbus are shown. The display covering the activities of *ñáñigo* and *brujería* (the latter the Cuban version of African voo-doo) is particularly effective.

The Museum of the City of Havana was established a few years ago in the old palace of the Lombillo family, one of the really fine colonial mansions that have been preserved on the Cathedral Plaza. It is in charge of Dr. Emilio Roig de Leuschsenring, the official historian of the city. Remains of the Siboneys and Tainos (as Cubans call the Arawaks) are at least as rich here as at the National Museum. Objects associated with the past of Havana are, of course, numerous and include furniture from the throne room of the Spanish captains general.

In the patio are to be seen various statues in marble and baser stone, from the old courthouse and from the Quinta de los Molinos where the captains general stayed in sum-mer. There is a *quitrín*, the typical fashionable carriage of the past century, given by the Menocal family. A large cabinet is devoted to relics of Martí. A lock of Simón Bolí-var's hair is treasured, and so is an authentic signature of his.

The revolutions against Spain and the War of Inde-pendence are amply covered. We find swords and pistols used in the last expedition of Narciso López, carbines from the Ten Years' War, and a twelve-pounder Hotchkiss quick-firer served at Victoria de las Tunas in 1897 by Fred-erick Funston, later a general in the United States Army. There are fragments of the U.S.S. *Maine*.

A small but excellent and growing library is maintained in connection with the Museum of the City of Havana. I found it most useful in the writing of this book.

Very interesting is the house where José Martí was born, and which is now a museum dedicated to him. It is a small two-story building, the ceilings low and the interior stairway narrow, the roof covered with red Spanish tiles, the courtyard constricted. This was the kind of house in which poor families lived during the last two centuries of the colonial period. It stands on the Calle Paula (now Leonor Pérez in honor of Martí's mother) near Egido, at a point that was overshadowed by the old city walls. The front room on the upper floor where the Apostle first saw the light on January 28, 1853, may not be entered by ordinary visitors; it is viewed across a barrier in the doorway. For the rest there are busts, tablets, cabinets containing objects associated with him, souvenirs, and books. The walls of the various rooms display photographs and framed documents by and about Martí.

At the end of the War of Independence the house was in a state of utter disrepair. Dr. Ramón L. Miranda, a devoted friend of Martí's, at once formed an organization to acquire and restore it. It took several years to accomplish this work. On February 24, 1909, the museum was finally opened by President José Miguel Gómez. Martí's mother, who lived to an advanced age, had died less than two years before. It is a place which most visitors to Havana overlook. The loss is theirs. Also in a sense a museum is the piously preserved stone quarry on the near edge of the Vedado, not far from the sea, where Martí worked in chains at the age of sixteen. More about this later.

Instituto No. 1, Havana's ranking high school and its oldest, Zulueta near Teniente Rey, houses the collection of birds made by Johannes C. Gundlach, the German who pioneered in Cuban ornithology a century ago. On the top floor is a reference library open to the public.

Cuba's national library, which contains more than 250,-000 items, including priceless historical documents, has occupied La Fuerza Castle for a number of years. The location is unsuitable. Only a few of the books are available on shelves, and long waits are often necessary before important volumes can be consulted. Recent governments have talked about the erection of a suitable building, but have failed to act. Now it seems likely that a plan of the kind will be carried through.

The library of the University of Havana is admirable. But the most modern library building in the city is that of the Sociedad Economica de Amigos del Pais, on Carlos III. After the founding of this organization by Captain General Luís de las Casas in 1793, it was commonly known as the Patriotic Society (see Chapter 9). Of late years it has devoted itself chiefly to free education, a cause aided by the enlarging and improving of its library.

The Instituto Cultural Cubano-Norteamericano, Calzada and H, Vedado, has made rapid progress in creating a public library named in honor of Martí and Lincoln. The Lyceum y Lawn Tennis Club, Calzada and 8, Vedado, maintains a good circulating library.

Chapter 27

THE MORRO AND SISTER FORTRESSES

THE MILITARY defensive fortresses of Havana were all given long, flowery names. The Morro, for instance, was El Castillo de los Tres Reyes del Morro—"The Castle of the Three Kings of the Morro"—the kings being those

who came to the cradle at Bethlehem, and Morro meaning
simply a headland, or promontory. The Cabaña was El
Castillo de San Carlos de la Cabaña. La Fuerza was originally the "royal" fortress, and La Punta was dedicated to
San Salvador. Atarés derives from one of the titles of the
Count de Ricla, the captain general under whom it was
started. Príncipe (prince, or sovereign) was named in honor
of a scion of the royal family, probably Carlos IV who was
heir apparent when it was completed.

The Morro was decided upon after the threatened attack
by Sir Francis Drake in 1585 (see Chapter 4). This had, as
a Spanish historian puts it, "enlightened the King, our
Lord Felipe II, surnamed the Prudent, to foresee, with his
great policy and incomparable penetration, that what was
then but a temptation to a few private corsairs would become in the future an object of desire to crowned heads."
The plans were drawn by the military engineer Juan Bau-
tista Antonelli. He copied a Moorish fortress then existing
at Lisbon, adapted it to the Havana headland, and finished
it in rough form by 1597. Changes later on improved the
design.

In part hewn out of the solid rock, it is an irregular
fortification, varying from 100 to 120 feet above the level
of the sea, and surrounded by moats 70 feet deep. The
lighthouse was erected by Captain General Leopoldo
O'Donnell in 1845, replacing an insignificant tower.

Visitors cross the harbor on the ferryboat and enter the
castle by an upward-sloping road bordered by poinciana
trees and tropical laurels, with adjoining hedges of cactus.
You come to a central court and from there are taken
through dark corridors on several levels. Some of the many
rooms are occupied, for part of the Morro is used as a
military school and there is a service personnel. Other

chambers are cells, ranging from fairly comfortable quarters to dungeons below the level of the water. A chute over the sea was intended for the disposal of garbage, but the story persists that under the Spaniards and under Machado the bodies of dead prisoners, and at times of living ones, were thrown down it to the waiting sharks.

At every turn you are impressed by the fact that this was a formidable defensive works, upon which Havana depended for its safety. It was captured only once, by the English in 1762 (see Chapter 7). Now it is completely outdated. A few salvos from modern battleships would bring it crumbling down, to say nothing of what bombardment from the air would do. Its long ramparts, with views of the sea and the city, constitute its most attractive feature. The eastward battery on the ocean side is called after that Captain Velasco who resisted Albemarle's troops so bravely. Low down by the waters of the harbor is the Battery of the Twelve Apostles, each of the guns being named for one of those who first rallied about Christ.

The fall of the Morro having demonstrated that alone it did not suffice, the long hill behind it and paralleling the harbor was crowned with linked fortifications. These constitute the Cabaña Castle. The project was vastly expensive. Its value, if any, was negative, for it has never been attacked and has never even fired a shot in war. Successive rulers have used it as a military jail and as a prison where political opponents could be kept hidden indefinitely, tried in secret and executed. Here is the Ditch of the Laurels, an empty moat where scores of Cuban patriots were shot during the Ten Years' War and the War of Independence. A line marked by the bullets of the firing squads can be traced for eighty-five feet along the wall. A bronze tablet sculptured in relief commemorates the endless tragedy of the

ditch, where most of the victims were young men taken
under arms. Here the poet Juan Clemente Zenea gave his
life.

The chief entrance to the Cabaña is on the land side, by
way of a drawbridge and sally port. It may be reached from
the city in launches which maintain a regular service from
three points, the fare being ten cents. Along with the
Morro, the Cabaña is not to be missed by those who have
the least curiosity about old fortresses. The two castles can
be done in a single trip, involving much walking, for they
are physically connected. The official tenant of the Cabaña
today is the artillery corps of Cuba. At nine o'clock every
evening a gun is fired in accordance with tradition. The
citizens of Havana set their watches by it. Formal national
salutes also are fired on the appropriate dates.

La Fuerza Castle, the most ancient of all, is on the west
side of the Plaza de Armas, and La Punta Castle stands
opposite the Morro. They are small compared with the
major works, and it is a long time since either of them
has been of defensive consequence. The first-mentioned replaced the original fort of Hernando de Soto (see Chapter
4), and has been sufficiently portrayed in these pages. It is
the temporary home of Cuba's national library.

La Punta has known its day of glory. There are cannon
on its walls which were not silenced by the British in the
siege of 1762 until the big guns of the captured Morro
were turned against them. It is now assigned to the Cuban
Navy as headquarters, with a garrison of marines. The
Naval Academy, where cadets are trained, is at Mariel in
Pinar del Rio province.

Virtually every traveler sees La Fuerza, and the majority
go to Morro and Cabaña. But Havana's two other castles,
Atarés and Príncipe, are seldom visited. The first is a war
college, with special postgraduate courses for promising

young infantry and artillery officers. The second has become a general penitentiary. I got permission to inspect both of them.

Atarés, which crowns a hill near the end of the harbor, is the farthest inland of the city's forts and commands a marvelous view of practically all Havana. It is triple-tiered, solidly bastioned, a jewel of a small castle in a good state of preservation. Atarés dates from the period immediately following the invasion by the English. Like the Cabaña, it never had to fight a foreign enemy but may have helped to deter aggressors. The slopes on all sides by which access may be had to it are so steep and crabbed that it is impossible to believe troops could have stormed them under fire. In the Machado revolution, however, mortars stationed below dropped shells upon the castle and made it untenable. Atarés was outdated.

The Spanish authorities had long regarded it as of subsidiary value only. When the Narciso López expedition was defeated in 1851, Colonel W. S. Crittenden of Kentucky and some fifty other prisoners, most of them North Americans, were taken to Atarés and executed there without a trial. A monolith halfway down one of the eastward slopes commemorates the tragedy. A similar monument pays tribute to Cuban martyrs in all the revolts against Spain—and in the Machado revolution.

Classrooms sectioned off in vaulted corridors, or made from bomb-proof (old-style) chambers with immensely thick walls and narrow windows, are full of students today. There is a military library. Texts on professional subjects are multigraphed on the premises, some of them emerging as thick bound volumes. The college seems to me a model of its kind. Those in charge respect the atmosphere of the place, which also should be noted to their credit. Gray stone walls have not been resurfaced, or rutted stairs leveled off with cement. Obsolete guns are kept in good condition, the tablets recording historical events carefully tended. Decorative trees improve the appearance of the lower reaches of the hill.

Príncipe Castle on its elevation north and a little to the east of Atarés is ideally placed for guarding the land approaches. It, also, has a magnificent view, taking in a wide sweep of the city and across to the ocean. The castle used to be surrounded by a moat, and according to legend tunnels connected it with several strategic points, including La Punta Castle. The moat has been filled in, and if the tunnels ever existed they have been sealed. So many structural changes have been made there, to adapt it to prison purposes, that its eighteenth-century characteristics have largely been lost. It can be visited only by permission of the Ministry of the Interior (Gobernación).

The modern conception of what a military headquarters should be is illustrated by Camp Columbia in Marianao. This center dates back to the United States occupation under Leonard Wood. Fulgancio Batista, during his first term in office, did more than any other Cuban president to develop it. The various buildings are considered models of military architecture.

Chapter 28

THE UNIVERSITY OF HAVANA

THE BUILDINGS grouped on rising ground at the end of San Lázaro which constitute the University of Havana are of different periods. This great seat of learning began to function on a modest scale in 1728 (see Chapter 6). It was then called a "royal and pontifical" university, and dedicated to San Gerónimo. In 1842 the ancient seminary of San Carlos was incorporated with it, and it was styled "royal and literary." Not until 1883, however, did it obtain recognition as the center of higher education for all Cuba. Its rector was in that year made chief of a "university district" comprising the six provinces of the island.

When Spanish rule ended in Cuba, the university at once benefited by important changes. Military structures on the present site, including cavalry barracks, were assigned to it by the United States authorities, and during 1899 all activities were transferred from Old Havana. The faculties of letters and sciences, law, and medicine and pharmacy, were retained and enlarged. Departments of pedagogy, architecture, and various branches of engineering were added. This was done under the direction of the eminent philosopher and historian Enrique José Varona, who had been appointed Secretary of Public Instruction, and who one day would be Vice-President of Cuba.

Other developments followed rapidly. Unsuitable buildings were replaced, often on a noble scale. After 1902 the republican government extended the university's holdings. Thus, the adjoining Quinta de los Molinos, summer residence of the Spanish captains general, was turned over.

Machado's dictatorship was a time of ordeal. Professors and students took a firmly democratic and patriotic stand. This led to acts of repression, and finally in December, 1930, the university for the first time in its history was closed by the government. It was not reopened until the fall of the regime in August, 1933. Another suspension occurred in 1935.

Today the university has reached heights of which its founders could not have dreamed. It has about 17,000 students and courses on almost every cultural and practical subject. It maintains a botanical garden. Natural history, anthropological and other museums exist within its walls. Its general library is of great distinction, and it has several specialized libraries. There is a stadium which seats 12,000 spectators.

The summer school, conducted on broad lines, is open to foreign students and is attended by many North Americans. It was founded in 1941. Two years later an institute of scientific investigations, and the broadening of studies was established. Then came a department of information, publications and cultural relations, which resulted in many valuable activities. A society of fine arts organizes activities such as exhibitions and concerts. The university's theater and its seminary of dramatic arts has staged both classic and modern plays.

Founded in 1946, the University of San Tomás de Villanova has been making good progress. It is backed by Catholics in the United States. The location is Avenida 5, in a development called the Reparto Biltmore, beyond Miramar.

Other universities are being planned for the capital, including a masonic one. They will meet special needs. They cannot in our times challenge the position of the University of Havana, which is able to enroll students for a basic charge of only $40 a year.

Though it is not a university, I wish to call attention here to the grand educational work in Spanish and English which is being done by the Instituto Cultural Cubano-Norteamericano, Calzada and H, in the Vedado. It was founded in 1943 by Cubans and North Americans; its library is dedicated jointly to José Martí and Abraham Lincoln. The general director is Dr. Herminio Portell Vilá, professor of American and modern history at the University of Havana, himself an established historian and a brilliant writer on many subjects. Languages and other subjects are taught at the Instituto. Anyone living in Havana may become a member and attend classes.

Chapter 29

MONUMENTS AND STATUES

HAVANA IS RICH in monuments, many of which have artistic merit. It is only proper to mention first the oldest memorial which has been preserved in Cuba. This is a stone tablet decorated with a cross and the head of an angel,

now to be seen on an interior wall facing the patio of the
Municipal Palace. It commemorates Doña María de Cepero
y Nieto, who in 1557, while praying in the parish church
of San Cristóbal which used to stand on that site, was
mortally wounded by the bolt of an harquebus carelessly
discharged outside. When the church was demolished 220
years later to make way for the palace of the captains general which has become the Municipal Palace, the Cepero
tablet was removed to the corner of Obispo and Officios. In
1914 it was placed in the National Museum. On the initiative of Dr. Roig de Leuchsenring, historian of the city, it
was returned to approximately its original position in 1937.

Carlos III. This appears to be the earliest monument of
any importance erected to a king or hero. The statue, which
is pleasing but not remarkable, is the work of Cosme de
Velázquez, though popularly attributed to Canova. It was
dedicated in 1803, being placed just outside the walls, and
removed in 1836 to its present location on the Paseo de
Carlos III.

La India, on the Prado side of the Plaza de la Fraterni-
dad. The beautifully modeled figure of the aboriginal wo-
man is regarded as an allegorical personification of the city.
The full name of this interesting monument, which stands
above a basin adorned with dolphins, is La Fuente de la
India o de la Noble Habana. Erected on its present site in
1837 by the Count of Villanueva, under the regime of
Tacón. In 1863 it was transferred to the middle of the
Parque Central, but twelve years later was shifted back.
Giuseppe Gaggini, an Italian, was the sculptor.

Christopher Columbus, in the patio of the Municipal
Palace. It is the work of J. Cucchiari, who designed it for
its present setting, where it was placed in 1862. Between
1870 and 1875 it adorned the Parque Central. Then, like
La India, it found its way home. As told in Chapter 23,

Columbus is also commemorated by a bust in front of El Templete, which incidentally is one of the few of him which show him bearded.

Fernando VII, in the Plaza de Armas. Erected to one of Spain's worst monarchs by Captain General Tacón in 1834. The statue, by Antonio Solá, has some artistic merit, which would appear to have been the only reason for preserving it after the independence of Cuba. There are mutilations inflicted by disgusted citizens, and the demand has often been made that it be sent to a museum and a statue of Carlos Manuel de Céspedes put in its place.

Miguel Cervantes, in the Plaza de San Juan de Dios. A tribute to the author of *Don Quijote*, by Carlos Nicoli.

General Francisco de Albear, in the Plazuela de Albear. Cuban-born and a great engineer, Albear constructed the waterworks at Vento, nine miles southwest of Havana, which till now have supplied the city. His monument, by the Cuban sculptor José Vilalta de Saavedra, was unveiled in 1895, the year the War of Independence started. The symbolical figure of Havana at its base offers a beguiling contrast with the Indian woman of La Noble Habana.

José Julián Martí, in the Parque Central. Also by Vilalta de Saavedra. Somewhat inferior artistically to the Albear, but of great historical significance as the first monument erected to Martí in Cuba. Its cost was met by public subscription. Dedicated on February 24, 1905, the tenth anniversary of the outbreak of the War of Independence, by President Tomás Estrada Palma and Generalissimo Máximo Gómez. The high reliefs about the base are worth noting.

The Student Martyrs of 1871, in the section of park named for them behind the Punta Castle. The monument takes the form of the piece of wall against which they were shot, now enclosed in a low temple of classic design. A suitable tablet describes the tragedy.

José de la Luz y Caballero, to the north of La Fuerza Castle, facing the Avenida de Céspedes. This monument to the early Cuban educator, philosopher, and patriot is by the sculptor Julien Lorieux, and was erected by public subscription in 1913.

General Antonio Maceo, in the Parque Maceo where Belascoain and San Lázaro meet. This is one of the two splendid, almost flamboyant, monuments erected so far to outstanding heroes of the War of Independence. An equestrian statue with supporting groups, by Domenico Boni, it was dedicated in 1916. It is the most imposing memorial in the Americas to a man of colored blood.

Generalissimo Máximo Gómez, facing the sea in the park in front of the National Palace. A companion piece in magnificence to the Maceo monument, and also consisting of an equestrian statue with supporting groups. It is by Aldo Gamba, and was unveiled in 1935.

Fountain of the Antilles, by Juan José Sicre, probably the best of young Cuban sculptors, in the park close to the Máximo Gómez monument. The supporting female figures are strongly modeled.

Maine Monument, in the waterfront park bearing the name of the ship, just beyond the Hotel Nacional. A delicate design consisting of two Corinthian columns, on which is perched an American eagle with outstretched wings. There are symbolical figures at the base. The sculptors Huertas and Cabarrocas utilized cannon and other relics from the *Maine* as decorations. The monument, erected in 1925, was destroyed in 1926 by a hurricane and reconstructed two years later. Immediately to the west of the Parque del Maine the new United States embassy is being built.

Juan Clemente Zenea, by Ramón Mateu, at the foot of

the Prado, facing Morro Castle. The figure of the poet who was executed by the Spaniards during the Ten Years' War is shown seated, with an attendant muse.

Dr. Carlos J. Finlay, on Belascoain near the Sagrado Corazón church. The statue of the originator of the mosquito theory in connection with yellow fever is by Ramón Mateu. There are supporting busts of Finlay's collaborators, including the North Americans, Major Gorgas and Dr. Lazear.

Plácido (Gabriel de la Concepción Valdés), the mulatto poet executed in the 1840's. It is by the Cuban sculptor Teodoro Ramos Blanco and stands in the Parque del Cristo.

· · *General Quintín Banderas,* in the Parque Trillo, the work of the Cuban sculptor Florencio Gelabert. Banderas was a notable Negro leader of irregulars in the War of Independence.

Alfredo Zayas, the fourth President, erected by himself behind the palace, though the inscription says that it was raised to him by "a grateful people." Cubans are sardonically amused by this monument and point it out to those visitors whom they trust have a sense of humor.

General Alejandro Rodríguez, on the Paseo, in the Vedado. He was the first *alcalde* (mayor) of Havana, elected in 1900 under Leonard Wood. The statue is by Giovanni Niccolini.

Mariana Grajales, the mother of the Maceos, by Teodoro Ramos Blanco. It stands at D and 23rd, Vedado, in a park named for her. This heroic mulatto woman's husband and all her sons, including the great Antonio, died for Cuba.

Francisco de Frias y Jacott, at Linea and K in the Vedado, of which residential district he was the founder. By the sculptor Domenico Boni.

Chinese Veterans' Monument, at Linea and L in the

Vedado. A fluted column of black stone, on the base of which the claim is made that no Chinese soldier in the revolutions against Spain ever deserted, or was ever a traitor.

Tomás Estrada Palma, on the Avenida de los Presidentes (Calle G). The first President of the republic.

José Miguel Gómez, by Giovanni Niccolini, at the far end of the Avenida de los Presidentes. A very elaborate monument to the second President. He is portrayed as a civilian, standing in front of a symbolic temple.

Victor Hugo, a bust by Juan José Sicre in the Parque Victor Hugo, H and 19th, Vedado.

There are also busts of Manuel de la Cruz, the poet and revolutionary patriot, at the Prado and the Parque Central; Miguel de Aldama, in the Plaza de la Fraternidad; America Arias, the wife of President José Miguel Gómez and the mother of President Miguel Mariano Gómez, behind the palace and also in the Plaza de Pasteur, Vedado; Cirilo Villaverde, the novelist, opposite the Angel Church; Gonzalo de Quesada, the friend of Martí and secretary of the New York junta; José Antonio Saco, the chief advocate of the abolition of slavery; Félix Varela, priest and patriot; Enrique José Varona, educator, philosopher, and statesman; General Enrique Collazo; Alexandre Pétion, the first President of Haiti; Simón Bolívar, the Liberator; Don Luís de las Casas, the best of the Spanish captains general of Cuba; Louis Pasteur, the great French scientist; William McKinley; Theodore Roosevelt; Leonard Wood; Andrew S. Rowan; and Woodrow Wilson.

With all these memorials, there are three salient omissions. Nowhere in Havana, though their names are used for streets and buildings, do we find monuments in the true sense of the term to Narciso López, Carlos Manuel de Céspedes, or Calixto García. Movements to fill the gaps have been started from time to time.

Chapter 30
THE COLON CEMETERY

AFTER VARIOUS burying grounds had proved inadequate—all of them of churchly origin—the Spanish authorities at last founded the Colón Cemetery, Zapata and 12,
situated roughly between Príncipe Castle and the Almendares River. This was in the latter part of the nineteenth
century. The designer, an architect named Calixto Loira,
had the mournful distinction of occupying its first grave.

There are cemeteries and cemeteries. This one is among
the most impressive in the world, ranking second only to the
modern necropolis of Rome according to many travelers.
The basis of such a judgment is the harmonious effect created by beautiful tombs and memorials, with a pervading
noble atmosphere deriving from the fact that the place is in
large part a national shrine. The gateway of Colón is itself
monumental, its arches well proportioned and above them
an effective crown of statuary; the limestone employed has
yellowed pleasingly.

A few yards down the main avenue you come upon the
tombs of the Generalissimo Máximo Gómez and his second
in command, Calixto García, facing each other. The Gómez
tomb is massive, surmounted by a dark stele, while that of
García is rather plain. Both heroes are accompanied by
members of their family. The note has been struck for

Colón Cemetery. A little farther on is the vault of the second President, José Miguel Gómez, where also reposes his lately deceased son, Miguel Mariano. It will be remembered that the younger man was removed from the presidency in 1936, after serving for only seven months (see Chapter 20). Admirers have affixed to the vault a tablet which quotes a law passed in 1950 to do posthumous justice to M. M. Gómez by annulling his removal.

Political controversy, as a matter of fact, finds plenty of expression in Colón. So does personal vanity. The tomb of Carlos Manuel de Céspedes the Younger, who was displaced in three weeks as provisional president after the fall of Machado, bears his portrait in relief and the words he uttered at the time: "Through me there will be no shedding of Cuban blood, or foreign intervention." The descendants of the Negro patriot of the War of Independence, Juan Gualberto Gómez (How that name Gómez recurs in Cuban history!) have seen fit to adorn his grave with a facsimile in bronze of a handwritten letter in which Martí addressed him as, "Beloved brother." As if the world needed to be reminded that the Apostle regarded all true patriots as brothers!

A striking contrast to the average is offered by the aristocratic third president of the republic. The Menocal family lot contains several simple white marble tombs, low and unadorned. Only one of them carries a name—General Menocal in small letters, and not a word more. It seems merely a courteous recognition of the point that the public has a legitimate claim to know where the dead leader lies.

The Count de Rivero, who published a newspaper, is symbolized as a knight in armor, with attendant damsels. There are many representations of Grief, and Death, and Fate, some of them extremely well wrought. Individuals, not always of the first rank of fame, are honored with life-size statues—a larger number with busts. Here and there the old-fashioned practice in Latin countries of setting up a sort of mortuary museum has survived. I noticed a grave which had a compartment in its headstone, faced with glass, containing a large photograph of a deceased grandmother and a selection of knick-knacks, including seashells, which presumably she had treasured in life.

Handsome collective monuments are to be seen. There is one to the martyred students of 1871, others to veterans of the War of Independence, to those who died in exile, and so forth. Easily the dominant memorial, as to size and flamboyance, is the one to the firemen who perished in a Havana conflagration on May 17, 1890. It was dedicated seven years later. A good deal of scorn has been directed at this monument, because it shouts down the tombs of so many eminent persons. Making allowances for the taste of the period in which it was built, however, it is not too bad. The tall column is surmounted by a figure of Sorrow, or Tragedy, supporting the body of a dead fireman, and at the four corners lower down there are statues of females in dramatic poses. Able sculptors contributed their work. The incidental flourishes, which ran even to the length of pendent bats, are certainly excessive.

Behind the Colón are to be found a Protestant cemetery and a Chinese cemetery.

Chapter 31

HOTELS AND CLUBS

THE HOTEL NACIONAL de Cuba is the finest in Havana, and naturally the most expensive. It was built about twenty-five years ago, but has been kept absolutely up to date. The site—on a bluff where the city proper joins the Vedado, with the long sweep of the Malecón on one hand and the Maine monument and plaza on the other—is incomparable. All its north windows look down upon the nearby ocean. It gets every breeze that blows. Morro Castle and the entrance to the harbor are in full view to the right. Apart from these things, it is a standard international hotel, and the sort of guest who sticks close to its comforts will not see much of typically Cuban life. Those who care about history will find the Nacional the more interesting for knowing that during the Machado revolution it was the center of dramatic events (see Chapter 19).

Next in rank as a luxury resort is the Sevilla-Biltmore, on the Prado at Trocadero. It is older than the Nacional, was *the* favored hotel of rich North Americans when Prohibition caused the first great rush of tourists to Havana, and is still first-rate. Many prefer it on account of its being at the center of the city.

Third place in the matters of size and attractiveness to the average tourist is shared by the Hotel Presidente, in the

196

Vedado, at Avenida de los Presidentes and Calzada, and the Hotel Plaza, downtown on Zulueta facing the Parque Central. The first-named has the advantages of quietude and closeness to the sea, the second of convenience for sightseeing and shopping.

Another kind of appeal is made by the few good hotels which have survived from the really old days, by which is meant the latter half of the nineteenth century. They have atmosphere, and in some cases have kept part of their colorful furnishings. The Inglaterra on the Parque Central is an example. This is the hotel which Joseph Hergesheimer described in his *San Cristóbal de la Habana*. It had been favored by rich Cubans and Spanish officers before the War of Independence, and it held its prestige under the republic until the tourist caravansaries were built. The Inglaterra had a great lobby, beautifully equipped and gorgeous with colored tiles. Its bedrooms also had paved floors; the ceilings were high and the long balconied windows shielded by Venetian blinds. The carved mahogany beds were draped at night with mosquito netting. Much of the lobby is now rented out for shops. The bedrooms have been modernized. Nevertheless, the house still has an air, and certain travelers swear by it.

The Pasaje and the Saratoga on the upper Prado fall into the same classification as the Inglaterra. Their lobbies appear even more desolate, being cluttered with varied commercial enterprises. The clientele at these two places is almost wholly Cuban.

The Ambos Mundos, equally archaic along different lines, is quite popular with North Americans. It is located at Obispo and Mercaderes, a tall building with practically no lobby but a roof garden that commands a wonderful view of the oldest part of Havana, the entrance of the harbor and the castles on the far shore. From the tables on one side of the restaurant up there you look straight down upon the flat *azotea* of the Municipal Palace. The late Thomas Barbour, the naturalist, was fond of the Ambos Mundos, as is Ernest Hemingway today.

Other hotels which can be recommended are the Alamac on Galiano, the Alcázar on Cardenas, the Azul on Presidentes, the Bristol on Amistad, the Catedral on San Ignacio, the Gran America on Industria, the Lincoln on Galiano, the Montserrat on Monserrate, the New York on Dragones, the Nueva Isla on Monte, the Ocean on the Malecón, the Packard on the Prado and Cárcel, the Parkview on Morro, the Perla de Cuba on Amistad, the Petit on Genios, the Regina on Industria, the Ritz on Neptuno, the Royal Palm on Industria, the San Carlos on Monserrate, the San Luís on Belascoain, the Siboney on the Prado, the Surf on the Malecón, and the Vedado on Calle 19.

Giving hotel rates in a book is of dubious wisdom, since rates change. And when they do they usually, alas, go up. In Havana there is a winter price and a summer price for those hotels that cater to tourists, the summer rates being considerably lower. In illustration I shall merely record that at one end of the scale the winter rates, European plan, of the Hotel Nacional in 1951 were: single, $18-20; double, $23-30. At the other end of the scale the Inglaterra charged: single, $6-8; double, $8-14. The Cuban Tourist Commission issues each season a complete list of the rates, and it is best to take that as a guide.

Havana is a city of clubs. The traveler is welcomed at even the exclusive ones, if properly introduced by one or two members, according to the rules of the club. A letter of introduction from a similar institution abroad, or a local sponsor, will suffice in many cases. For games such as tennis and golf, for swimming and general entertainment, tourists depend largely upon the clubs. The following are some of the more celebrated and hospitable places:

The American Club, Prado and Virtudes. It was founded during the administration of Cuba by the United States after the War of Independence. The membership is composed mainly of resident North Americans, but a fair number of Cubans belong to it. A social club equal to the finest in New York or Washington.

The Lyceum & Lawn Tennis Club, Calzada in the Vedado. A women's cultural center with wide activities, including a good library.

Havana Biltmore Yacht and Country Club, in suburban Jaimanitas. Spacious grounds and excellent golf links. The atmosphere is almost as North American as it is Cuban.

Vedado Tennis Club, Calzada and 12; Country Club de la Habana, Marianao; Club Nautico, Marianao; Casino Deportivo de la Habana; Casino Español; Rotary Club, Hotel Nacional; Union Club, Malecón near San Lázaro.

There are several chess clubs, of which the most important are the Club de Ajedrez ("chess") de la Habana, established in 1885; and the Club Capablanca, founded five or six years ago to honor the memory of the great Cuban chess champion of the world, the late José Raúl Capablanca.

Strictly Cuban and visited by tourists only for the sake of inspecting the buildings are the Centro Gallego, the Centro Asturiano (to both of which references have been made elsewhere in this book), the Asociación de Dependientes, the Hijas de Galicia, the Asociación Canaria, and the Centro Castellano. They are amazing organizations, which for dues averaging $2.50 a month provide their members with educational facilities, medical attention, social entertainment, and a large number of other benefits. The active memberships of the three leading societies were given in

1951 as 52,051 for the Centro Gallego, 78,156 for the Centro Asturiano, and 72,719 for the Dependientes.

Chapter 32

THE CASINO AND THE LOTTERY

GAMBLING IS a major passion among Cubans. As noted in the historical section of this book, it always has been so. Moralists regard it as the country's chief vice. Serious efforts to stamp it out have been made from time to time, but these have never been fully successful nor maintained for long. The Casino Nacional, Marianao, built about thirty years ago and leased as a concession, has had curious ups and downs. There have been periods when it was the only legal gambling house in the capital, others when it has faced unlimited competition, and others when it has been ordered to close its doors. It enjoys no monopoly at present, but its semi-official standing draws most of the big money to its tables.

There are two buildings in beautiful grounds, the smaller one being known as the Summer Casino or *Casino de la Playa*. The fountain at the entrance of the grounds is deservedly popular. Around the rim of the white marble basin dance eight nude nymphs, while seated female figures, also naked, support the basin in the role of caryatids. When the fountain is not playing, the clear waters of the pool carry a reflection of the sculpture in reverse. The piece is the work of Aldo Gamba, the Italian who did the Máximo Gómez monument.

Both the large and small casinos are social centers, with restaurants, bars, ballrooms, and floor shows, as well as gambling halls. Most years the principal building operates only during the winter season—December to March, inclusive. The lesser one fills in for the rest of the year. To go to either of them you are not obliged to play, but the majority of patrons simply cannot resist the temptation. Tourists feel they have come to the Monte Carlo of the West Indies, and that it would be a bit absurd to leave without indulging in a flurry.

Roulette is the perennially favored game of chance, its wheel the medium of sheer luck. It is closely pressed by baccarat and chemin-de-fer, which resemble each other. In straight baccarat any number of players, usually eighteen, oppose a banker for the house. The object is to hold cards totaling nearer to nine than those of the banker. In chemin-de-fer a bidder takes the bank, playing against all the others until he loses, or until he chooses to relinquish it.

Craps and electric poker are well liked. The last-mentioned is a machine that drops cards into a display rack when buttons are pushed. You push five buttons and you get a poker hand. If you have one pair or better you may draw to the hand. The pay-off is on two pairs or better, at various odds. The house has an edge of 10 per cent in electric poker, yet people continue to play it ardently.

Many other games are offered at the Casino, some of them the fads of a single season. The greenhorn will make no mistake if he sticks to roulette, the functioning of which is perfectly clear, as well as dramatic. That the Casino conducts its games honestly has never been questioned.

All gambling establishments encourage the spreading of

luck stories because they are good for business. The one
that I heard in Havana and told in my *Lands of the Inner
Sea* is so remarkable that it deserves to be repeated, though
with no guarantee that it should be taken for gospel. It
appears that a quiet little American woman in the season
of 1928-29 lingered near a roulette wheel for a while, then
placed a dollar bill on a full number. She won at thirty-five
to one, a thing that happens every day. The woman let her
winnings ride, but on another number, and won again:
$1,260. Spectators gathered about her and urged her to
pyramid. She hesitated nervously, divided the amount and
staked $630. She cleaned up once more and there was wild
excitement. Was this to be the feminine counterpart of
"the man who broke the bank at Monte Carlo?" But she
cashed in her chips, hurried from the Casino with a total of
$22,680, and was not seen there again.

The most astonishing part of the story is its sequel. A few
months afterward, another American woman entered the
Casino, walked right up to the same roulette wheel, and
successfully backed three full numbers in sequence. No one
remembers whether these were the original bettor's numbers; presumably they were. The second woman left as
hurriedly and as finally as the first had done. Of course, the
Casino authorities conducted an inquiry. They found that
the two women were both schoolteachers and came from
the same state, though not the same town. It is to be in-
ferred that they knew each other, and that upon learning
of the first one's luck the second had come to Havana for
the sole purpose of trying to repeat the coup. Their names
were not made public.

Gambling makes its widest appeal through the national
lottery, which has attained enormous proportions since it
was founded early in the nineteenth century, suppressed
after the War of Independence, and revived under Presi-

dent José Miguel Gómez. There are now drawings every week with a top prize of $100,000, and hundreds of consolations scaling down to $100. At Christmas and on certain special occasions there is a grand prize of $300,000. It has been calculated that against each 25,000 tickets issued the customers have 1,429 chances to win some kind of prize. No other game exists in which the bank (in this case, the state) is certain of so high a percentage of the money risked. Yet mankind is unfailingly allured by it.

Few full tickets are bought in Cuba, for their price is not less than $20. The ticket is divided into a hundred fractions, nominally at twenty cents but retailing at twenty-five cents for ordinary drawings, and relatively more for the grand Christmas drawing. Almost everyone takes a chance at the minimum figure. Others buy blocks of fractions, quarter-tickets, or half-tickets. It is common for groups of workers in offices or shops, to subscribe each week for shares in a full ticket. Every conceivable system is followed in connection with supposedly lucky numbers. Despite the fact that hawkers of tickets swarm the streets and invade the buses, there is ample scope for sales at fixed locations. In a long arcade on Galiano, there is even a lottery market with many dealers whose specialty is finding and furnishing the exact "hunch" numbers the purchasers want.

The drawings take place at 2 P.M. on Saturday in headquarters at Amargura and Cuba. Orphans from the Casa de la Beneficencia, an institution that is in part supported by lottery funds, act as the agents of fortune. After the huge container filled with numbers has been rotated, an orphan picks a number blind and simultaneously releases a ball which indicates the value of the prize it has won. The ceremony goes on for hours. It is open to the public.

Lottery luck tales are still more numerous than those told about the Casino. There was the rich young man years ago who was twitted by a group of friends on the eve of the Christmas drawing, because he was the only one who did not hold a chance. It was a minute or so to the deadline, but he sent out a messenger who encountered an old woman peddler going home and bought a full ticket from her. That ticket won the *premio gordo:* $300,000. The young man used most of it to treat the entire group of friends who had been with him to a round trip to Paris. It happens to be a true story.

Quite recently, a man who had been in the habit of buying the same number week after week from the same dealer slipped up through being out of town, then was aghast to read that the number in question had drawn the top prize. He returned sadly to Havana, opened the drawer of his desk —and found the ticket staring at him. The dealer had brought it as usual and had left it, trusting his old customer to pay. That one, also, is true.

Not content with the drawings of the lottery itself, thousands of persons play a numbers racket called the *bolita.* Even the receipts given for each fare paid on the buses carry numbers, and if you hold one that corresponds with a winner in the national lottery you collect a prize.

Chapter 33
PARKS, BEACHES, AND PLAYGROUNDS

SPANISH COLONIAL cities, and especially walled ones, had little space to devote to parks. There was a main plaza, in which sometimes there would be trees and beds of flowers. Other public breathing spots were small and almost invariably paved. The patios of private houses served in lieu of parks. True to form, Old Havana offers us only the Plaza de Armas from early days. The Plaza de la Catedral and Plaza de San Francisco are simply cobblestoned areas in front of churches. The Plaza del Cristo and Plaza de San Juan de Dios are true parks in miniature, but much more recent. The so-called Plaza Vieja—though it is not so old as the Plaza de Armas—between San Ignacio and Inquisidor, has been until lately just a crossroads for traffic; it is now being made over. The landscaping of part of the waterfront is an improvement dating from yesterday.

Numerous references in previous chapters to the Plaza de Armas have pretty well covered the subject. As its name implies, it was originally regarded as chiefly a site for military display. Its form has been altered more than once. Ancient prints show it crossed by driveways, while at other periods it was given over to shaded footpaths where ladies and men of fashion strolled in opposite directions to observe one another demurely. The Plaza de Armas seems

205

never to have been an outstandingly beautiful square. It has been the scene of historic events, however, and much pageantry, since the palace which housed the Spanish captains general faces upon it. On the northwestern corner is El Templete which commemorates the first mass said in Havana, and to the left looms the picturesque mass of La Fuerza Castle in which the national library is temporarily installed.

Though they serve merely to decorate open spaces, this is as good a place as any to mention the sections of the old city walls which have been preserved. One overgrown with vines and including a tiny watchtower, is directly in front of the Presidential Palace. Far from spoiling the view, it integrates the palace most effectively with the past of the city. Another fragment of wall is to be seen between Monserrate and Zulueta, beside Instituto No. 1. The largest, near the railroad station on Egido, is called the Baluarte del Angel and bears a recently affixed map in bronze of ancient Havana within its bulwarks.

The Parque Central, an unimaginative name but an accurate one in this case, is at the very heart of Havana, between Old and New. It was formerly named after Isabel II of Spain. The Prado extends along its western side. Two large hotels face it, as do the magnificent buildings of the Centro Gallego and the Centro Asturiano. The Capitol looms just to the south. Vilalta Saavedra's statue of Martí is the only monument in the Parque Central, which is thick with laurel trees trimmed formally. Royal poincianas grow there also. A small, intimate landscaped square, known to everyone who has visited Havana.

Beyond the Capitol is the Plaza de la Fraternidad, originally the Campo de Marte, a military parade ground. The celebrated statue of La India stands at one corner. Under the republic it was decided to dedicate this park to the Pan-

American idea. A ceiba tree was planted at its center in soil brought from all the independent American countries and enclosed with a handsome circular bronze fence. This was on the occasion of the Sixth Pan-American Conference, which was held in Havana in 1926. Busts of Simón Bolívar, Abraham Lincoln, and other supreme figures were subsequently spaced throughout the park.

Broadening in from the Malecón at the Calzada de Belascoain is the Parque Maceo, site of the equestrian statue to the great mulatto general. The park is not landscaped, but has a reflecting pool with a fountain, a playground for children, and numerous benches. The San Lázaro tower at one end was built in 1556 as a vantage point from which to watch for hostile sails. Close by, on Hospital near Infanta, is the San Lázaro stone quarry where Martí worked in chains when sentenced for sedition at the age of sixteen. The quarry and the cloistral garden in front of it contain objects related to the Apostle. Officially named the Rincón Martiano, it is, after the birthplace house, the most intimate of his shrines in Havana.

A few blocks farther down, covering two squares on the waterfront in the Vedado, we find the Parque José Martí, a juvenile playground still better equipped than the one in the Parque Maceo.

In line with modern city planning, there are many adequate parks in the Vedado and nearby suburbs. La Tropical and La Polar breweries maintain recreation gardens on the outskirts which are in effect public parks; La Tropical is perhaps the better known, because of the large fetes that have been held there.

The Botanical Gardens, which comprise the grounds of the Quinta de los Molinos, summer home of the Spanish captains general, are now run by the University of Havana. The entrance is on Carlos III. An unusually fine collection of regional trees, shrubs, and flowers has been developed. The original garden was on the site of the Capitol and was shifted to the Quinta when it was displaced by a railroad station that preceded the Capitol.

Comparatively new is the Zoological Park at 26th and Aldecoa, in the Vedado. According to the last count it contained some 1,200 animals. The sculptured group of deer climbing a rock at the main gateway is much admired. There is a "monkey town," where the freedom of the simians is but slightly restricted. This zoo may be reached from downtown or the Vedado by bus routes numbered 26, 27, and 79.

La Concha, at La Playa de Marianao, is the only public beach in Havana. All the others have been pre-empted by clubs. A small charge is made at La Concha. Four bus routes—30, 32, I-1, and U-4—connect with it. The need for developing suitable waterfront land for the use of the people is recognized. Plans are afoot to create public beaches farther west along the Gulf of Mexico, and on the northern shore beyond Morro Castle.

Chapter 34
RACING: BOTH HORSES AND DOGS

HAVANA WAS always a natural setting for horse racing, since its citizens like to bet. Yet the sport developed slowly there. Toward the end of Spanish rule it was practiced on a small scale. The republic did nothing to foster it until the presidency of Menocal, when liberal gambling concessions attracted capital from the United States and Oriental Park was founded. The track, located in Marianao, has become one of the most famous in the Americas. The Jockey Club associated with it is a luxurious resort, which not only has the best stand for watching the races but offers general gambling facilities second only to those of the Casino Nacional. Its cuisine, orchestra, and floor shows are excellent.

Oriental Park is beautifully located against a rich tropical background, with royal palms in the distance, a hedge of giant bamboos around the far reaches of the mile-long course, and flowerbeds close at hand ablaze with color. The grandstand seats 5,000 persons. A novelty here is that you may place bets either at parimutuel windows, or with bookmakers who give about the same odds. I was informed that the public prefer the bookmakers, because of the chance occasionally to pick up a bargain that is not governed by the wagers of other patrons.

The winter season runs from December to March, inclusive, when there ordinarily are daily races except on Mondays and Fridays. With little or no interruption there follows a long summer season, offering meets on Tuesdays, Thursdays, Saturdays, Sundays, and all holidays. The Government admits race horses and their paraphernalia into the country free of duty if they are to be run at Oriental Park. This has simplified the bringing of star attractions from the United States, indeed has made Havana a unit of the North American circuit. Horse racing is good for Cuba's tourist business, not to mention the fact that it attracts big money unrelated to tourism. The present Batista administration has indicated that it will give wider support.

Though the Jockey Club is selective, it is not exclusive.

It is simply a device to furnish space, comfort, and special entertainment for those who can afford to pay. There are about 16,000 regular members, but any well-dressed, well-behaved person can buy an entrance ticket at some five times the cost of grandstand admission, or obtain a clubhouse membership for the season. Señor Mario García Herrera, the social manager, told me that the day of the plunger, the heavy gambler, appears to have passed—perhaps temporarily. But a volume of modest betting by the public at large maintains Oriental Park as a successful track. There is no other of its standard in Cuba.

The distance from the Havana hotels being considerable, most visitors go out to Oriental Park by car. However, it is possible to reach it by several bus routes which pass by way of the Parque Central. Look for the sign *Hipódromo* in front of the bus.

Greyhound racing is a brand-new and increasingly popular sport in Havana. As it is staged at night, it does not seriously cut into the attendance at horse races. The arena is located opposite the La Concha beach, Miramar, at the foot of the avenue that previously was best known for the resorts called La Fritas. Some of the latter were demolished to make way for the arena, which inevitably has changed the district's atmosphere.

Jerry Collins, the impresario of the dogs, should more formally be described as manager of the Havana Kennel Club. He has introduced to local sport the tastes and methods of Miami, with the difference that open and unrestricted gambling adds to the fun here. The lightning-fast heats and quick turnover of bets delight the Cubans.

Chapter 35
GAMES: JAI-ALAI AND BASEBALL

JAI-ALAI IS probably Havana's most popular game, as distinguished from a sport. There can be no doubt that this was true in the past, but some authorities say that it has been outdistanced by baseball. It remains extremely popular, and its star performers earn record incomes. Seven thousand dollars a month was not thought too much to pay Emilio Equiluz a few years ago. Jai-alai is a Basque game, the meaning of the name in that tongue being roughly, "gay fiesta." In Spanish it is often called *pelota* (ball). The building in which it is played is a *frontón*, though the strict meaning of that word is the main wall of a handball court. Jai-alai, in fact, is a variety of handball, the fastest that has ever been developed.

The court is an oblong, and if of standard size is 210 feet long and 36 feet wide, the floor of cement and the walls of granite. There are three walls, the front one against which the scoring is done, a long wall to the left of the players, and a rear wall. The fourth side is screened with wire netting, behind which are boxes, open benches, and a gallery for the public. The protection afforded by the wire is essential, for the ball travels with such speed and force that it could kill a person. It is like a solid, enlarged golf-ball, but of course smooth.

Several variations of jai-alai are recognized, but the game most often played is between two-men teams of Blancos (whites) and Azules (blues). The men wear strapped to the right hand and wrist a narrow, curve-shaped *cesta* ("basket") about two feet long, which is in effect an extension of the palm. By means of this a terrific momentum in delivering the ball is obtained. The player who starts off bounces the ball on the floor, catches it in his cesta and serves it against the front wall. Then it is caught on the fly or first rebound by a member of the other side. It may carom from the left or rear walls without its counting against the player, as only the bound on the floor is considered. The ball passes furiously between the teams until a player misses or strikes out of bounds. This scores a point for the other side.

Any stipulated number of points may constitute a game; in Havana it is generally twenty-five or thirty points. Betting agents stationed in front of the lowest tier of seats accept wagers not only before the play starts, but at any subsequent stage of the game. The odds vary widely, and with startling rapidity. A favorite team ahead 15 to 11 may be quoted at 5 to 1—only to become short-enders a few minutes later, because the other side has rallied. If the betting-agent cannot reach a customer readily, he tosses him a hollow ball. The amount of the bet is placed in the ball and thrown back to the agent. It seems a casual way to risk money, but all is conducted with scrupulous honesty.

Jai-alai stars are the idols of their public. They are required to be graceful as well as adroit, and the opportunities of the game lend themselves to grace. A favorite who has bungled is quite likely to bury his face in his arms for a moment or sob openly; no Latin would sneer at this display of emotion, which is admired, rather, as proof of sincerity and artistic temperament.

There are two great frontóns in Havana. At the Frontón Jai-Alai, Concordia 556, games are held every evening except Mondays and Fridays. The Frontón Havana-Madrid, Belascoain 803, puts on games every afternoon at 3:00 P.M., and on Mondays and Fridays in the evening. Most of the players, incidentally, are Spaniards.

Baseball has enjoyed a tremendous vogue for years. This has been largely due to the fact that many of the major league clubs in the United States found it agreeable to do their training in the environs of Havana. Local youngsters caught the fever, dreamed of the game as a road to celebrity and cash. A Cuban, Adolfo Luque, performed brilliantly on a world's-championship team, and he has had successors. But to call baseball Cuba's national game, as is often done in print, seems to me an exaggeration. Havana has a professional league composed of four teams. It attracts crowds during the season (October to February) when games are held nightly. On Sundays the teams meet in the afternoon, as well as at night. Amateur championships are disputed during the summer months.

But I am convinced that baseball would wither in Cuba if it were not for the element of gambling, freely permitted here. The pious horror of North Americans at betting on baseball is something the Havanese do not understand, or want to understand.

The principal diamonds where the clubs clash are in the Grand Stadium of Havana, between Monte and the Rancho Boyeros highway; and the stadiums in the gardens of the Tropical and Polar beer companies. The stadium of the University of Havana is open only to amateur teams.

Chapter 36

WHEN THE COCKS FIGHT

COCKFIGHTING, now, is a sport rather than a game, and in Cuba it attains the dimensions of a national hobby. Havana has cockfight clubs which hold mains for members only, though the entree is liberally extended to strangers. Many of the enthusiasts raise their own birds, and they are as impassioned over the fine points of breeding and training as any race horse owner could be. The same ardor is to be found among the patrons of the public *vallas* (cockpits). Newspapers have cockfight columns, in which performances are discussed by able critics. Champions earn island-wide fame and, if placed on the market, command very high prices; many have pedigrees dating back for generations.

Some of the best strains were originally crossed with English fowls, or that is the tradition. The type is called Inglés. There is also a fine breed known as Jerezano, descended from birds imported from the sherry-wine district of southern Spain. The purely Cuban varieties are supposed to be inferior, but every year they furnish a quota of sturdy fighters. There is an interchange on a small scale with fanciers in Mexico and Florida.

The *valla* is a ring, or pit, enclosed by a breast-high wooden wall and with sawdust on the earth. The choice seats are located at ground level around the arena. Benches

214

rise in circular tiers to a conical roof. Usually there is no exterior wall. The *valla* has a backyard where there are coops for the birds entered in the current main, or possibly in a longer tournament. They chortle and crow incessantly. The privileged addicts go and look them over before the show starts. A gamecock trimmed down for action has had his comb pared of excrescences on to which an opponent might hang, and the long feathers plucked from his neck and thighs. He is rarely allowed to use his own spurs; these are filed, and the cured spurs of another bird are placed over them and taped to his legs. According to the jargon of the sport, the "cold" spurs inflict a more damaging wound than would be the case with the "hot" spurs of the living cock. If the rules of the contest provide for it, steel spurs may be substituted with the object of obtaining more swift and deadly results.

When the two adversaries have been inspected and weighed, they are brought to opposite sides of the pit. Sometimes they are allowed to see each other, while held tightly, so that they may work up a rage. This is just drama, for they need no stimulus. Two tin cages without bottoms are lowered on a cord to the ground, a cock is placed in each one, and at a signal from the referee the cages are lifted simultaneously. The birds throw themselves upon each other. Needless to say, the betting has been furious, and as in jai-alai it continues with shifting odds throughout each match.

Anglo-Saxons profess to find the cockfight revolting on the grounds of cruelty. Those from the puritanic northern belt are doubtless sincere about it, but most Southerners are "fans" even if they come from a state where the sport is illegal. In my opinion the element of cruelty is slight, if it exists at all. Gamecocks are incurably pugnacious. They enjoy fighting, and if they did not battle in the pit they would find a way to do so outside it. The argument that they perpetrate crude butchery is shallow, too. The varying technique employed by different cocks is fascinating and often astonishing.

I recall a main I attended in Havana where the first two birds were an ordinary-looking speckled fellow, and a flashy, handsome white cock. The public seemed to know little about them and took the obvious course of supporting the white in the betting. All the early points were scored by the white. The speckled actually ran away. Time and again, he scuttled around the pit, and when almost overtaken he turned and buried his head under his opponent's wing. It was like clinching in a boxing match. The white would exert a great effort, shake him off and try to nail him with beak and spurs. But the speckled would be gone, weaving and sliding, his body crouched.

The spectators did not know what to make of it. The majority of them hooted and yelled that the cowardly bird should be disqualified. A few had their doubts and started to bet on him. That fight lasted for twenty minutes, a phenomenal length in the cockpit. Suddenly the speckled turned and attacked with positive artistry. He was much the fresher of the two. It became clear that he had deliberately saved his strength and induced the other to wear himself out. He cut down the white with half a dozen strokes and killed him.

Next on the program was a contest that took three minutes. The two cocks were armed with spurs that had been sharpened to needle points, and both of them were birds that practiced direct tactics. They sprang into the air, facing each other, lashing out with both legs. They were like fencers rather than boxers. One of them broke through his antagonist's guard and pierced his head with a dagger-like spur. It was all over. A more complete contrast between this fight and the preceding one could not be imagined.

The most interesting public cockpit is the Valla Habana on Agua Dulce Plaza, in the suburb of Jesús del Monte. It is easily reached by bus. Mains occur on Saturday, Sunday, and Monday in the afternoon. Ringside seats are three dollars, a perch on one of the bare benches of the gallery from fifty cents to a dollar. That, at least, is what they charge tourists now that the place has become well known. A main in nearby Guanabacoa, where they have very good ones, can be seen on a Sunday for a dollar, ringside. The best private organizations are the Club Gallistico de la Habana, and the Club Gallistico Moderno in the Vedado. There are similar clubs throughout Cuba. They often challenge one another and hold great meets.

The bullfight, abolished at the end of the War of Independence, was legalized in 1947 with the rules modified to forbid the killing of the bull. But the public would have none of it. When a contest was announced there were mob demonstrations against it as a "Spanish vice," and the idea had to be dropped.

Chapter 37
THEATERS, LEGITIMATE AND OTHERWISE

As is the case throughout the world, "live" or legitimate drama has been pretty well dispossessed in Havana by the cinema. The Nacional, Payret, Martí, and

Principal de la Comedia are the only dignified theaters which still cling to the older art, and even they often show movies for one reason or another. The Campoamor, formerly a house of some pretensions, divides its bookings about equally between musical comedy and motion pictures. This state of affairs is not pleasing to lovers of the stage. It is particularly deplored that the splendid *Nacional*, once the Tacón, which is now incorporated in the Centro Gallego building on the Parque Central, tends more and more to be used as a concert hall and has lost its significance and atmosphere.

A movement to remedy this by creating a real national theater has been launched, with official backing. Part of the profits from one of the lottery drawings in the spring of 1952 was pledged to the fund, and each fraction of a ticket carried the statement.

The *Payret*, upper Prado facing the Capitol, is an old house lately reconstructed and made to look too modern if anything. It imports operettas from Europe and the Americas. But it frequently offers a movie, with singing or dancing stars before and after. The ancient devotees of both the Nacional and the Payret must stir uneasily in Colón Cemetery. For it was to the Nacional that grand opera and the classic drama used to come, while the Payret was the home of the sparkling light comedy typical of Latin capitals fifty years ago.

The *Martí*, Zulueta and Dragones, has been consistently the home of operetta and vaudeville, mostly brought from Spain. This theater used to be called the Irijoa, and in 1901 it was the scene of independent Cuba's first constituent convention. For that reason it was given the name of the patriot, José Martí.

The *Principal de la Comedia*, Animas and Zulueta, specializes in the showing of Spanish plays. On occasions,

when it would otherwise be dark, this attractive old downtown house is utilized by groups comparable to the "little
theater" movement in the United States.

The *Campoamor*, Industria and San José. It has been
mentioned above, and further comment is unnecessary.

Among the multitudinous cinema theaters, the following
deserve to be singled out:

Alkázar, Consulado and Virtudes. An oldish house lately
reconditioned.

Negrete, on the Prado opposite the Sevilla-Biltmore
Hotel. It shows chiefly pictures made in Spanish-speaking
countries.

Fausto, Prado and Colón.

Plaza, Prado 210.

Encanto, Neptuno between Consulado and Industria.
Sometimes offers live acts.

America and *Radio Cine*, standing side by side on Galiano between Neptuno and Concordia. These two large,
first-class houses are among the best erected in Havana to
show moving pictures.

Warner, 23rd and L, Vedado. Also a thoroughly modern,
comfortable house. "Name" bands and featured performers "in person."

Riviera, 23rd 507, Vedado.

Trianon, Linea 706, Vedado.

Blanquita, Avenida 1, Miramar. One of the largest theaters in the world. Offers stage attractions along with pictures.

Miramar, 86th and 5th, Miramar.

Atlantic, between 10th and 12th, Vedado.

Astral, Infanta and San José.

Rex and *Duplex*, San Rafael between Industria and
Amistad. Decidedly one of the most elaborate newsreel
combinations to be found anywhere. The Rex offers only

actualities, spiced with a travelogue and an animated cartoon. The Duplex features an artistic film play, bolstered by news. The two theaters have a common lounge stocked with magazines, where their patrons may read and smoke as long as they choose.

Auditorium, Calzada and D, Vedado, owned by a great musical organization which calls itself the "Pro-Arte," is where grand opera, philharmonic orchestras, and ballet usually appear.

Anfiteatro ("Amphitheater") Nacional, on Puerto midway between La Fuerza and La Punta castles, is run by the state. Free concerts by municipal, military, and other official bands are given several times a week.

Chapter 38
NIGHT LIFE IN HAVANA

THE CUBAN NOVELIST Felix Soloni wrote in his *Mersé* (1926) that Havana was not a city for night-roving. The few who stayed awake after one A.M., according to him, were "watchmen, street cleaners, artists suffering from insomnia, bored journalists, chauffeurs, and policemen. Those who drive dull care away by getting drunk on the fourth glass cause a mild scandal and either land in the police station or wander home. And nothing more! This, mind you, occurs only in the vicinity of the Parque Central;

around both Old and New Havanas, nothing. The cabarets are in the outskirts, and their clientele is always the same." He conceded that American tourists, whom he found quite ridiculous, did manage to stir up a little excitement.

It may have been that dull in the middle 1920's at the start of the Machado regime, though I doubt it. Havana knew how to amuse itself lustily in earlier periods (see Chapters 10 and 15), and certainly is not behindhand to-day. Soloni's basic contention, however, is that the average resident goes to bed early, which is true of all Latin cities, including Paris. The night-hawk is a special variety of bird. Some Havanese go by choice where the tourist goes, while others pursue pleasure in ways of which the tourist never hears.

The lures are eternally the same: dancing, and entertainment by dancers, singers and exhibitionists of one kind and another; sports on which betting is allowed, and various games of chance; drinking, with incidental eating; and prostitution. Havana offers all these things, ranging from the luxurious to the cheap and sordid.

The sidewalk cafés of the upper Prado, opposite the Capitol, offer a pleasant start for a dip into night life. There is nothing sensational about them. They are extensions of long-established cafés, such as the El Dorado and the Saratoga. Most have orchestras, with featured singers or an occasional solo dance act. I remember an all-girl orchestra which was so popular with the male customers that it had to be enclosed in a glass cage; anyhow, that was the publicity story. The drinks are reasonably priced for resorts of the kind, which in New World cities are burdened by ground taxes. Personages of the theater and sports favor these open-air cafés, but sooner or later everybody comes.

Genial old Don Gabriel Camps, a journalist and man

about town, who revived the custom on the upper Prado some twenty-five years ago, put it to me as follows: It was a commonplace to extol the joys of watching the world go by, he declared, but what about the satisfaction of being seen by the world as one lolled in a fashionable spot? Much might be said, too, for the advantage of being able to tell at a glance who were the patrons of a given café without having to enter and partly commit oneself to taking a seat. If you noted a boring acquaintance who was likely to buttonhole you, why you saluted him vaguely and passed on. Somewhere else you were sure to observe a friend with whom you did want to talk.

After the open-air cafés, the logical progression is to the night bars or the night clubs. They are very different institutions in Havana. The first offer no theatrical entertainment, but are frequented by girls playing the role of hostesses whose obliging ways are more candid than those of their sort in the United States. The night clubs have elaborate programs, beginning usually at a late hour, whereas the night bars function from cocktail time on. So give the latter an initial look. Escorted ladies are admitted, though their presence is regarded as slumming and causes a certain uneasiness. My suggestion is intended for men.

The blocks on Virtudes closest to the Prado on either side are downtown headquarters for this kind of bar. Names need not be mentioned. No one could miss the places with their garish electric signs, the clustering of hopeful taxis, and the policemen seated in doorways who advise tourists if asked and settle disputes amicably. The typical bar is air-conditioned, well furnished, and has a small backroom for dancing to juke-box music. Drinks are at moderate prices. The girls constitute the main attraction. They are under police control, will sit beside an unaccompanied man and ask him to buy a round, but will excuse themselves politely if he says no. Any one of them may be taken from the premises. To bring that about is their object. The house scrupulously protects the right of the customer to be a mere looker-on, however, and does not hurry him over his drinks.

Havana night clubs follow the international pattern, but are decidedly more colorful than in most countries. The Spanish dance, which is an art form of a high order, is responsible for this, with the potent aid of the variations that have been developed through the years in Cuba.

The principal hotels and the Casino Nacional, which is the Monte Carlo of the Caribbean, have night club attractions. Indeed, there are times when the Casino captures so many of the good acts that it claims pre-eminence. Notable among the independent spots are the following:

Tropicana, occupying a former mansion on the Avenida Truffin, Buena Vista suburb in the direction of Marianao. The gardens here are charming, the food excellent, and the professional entertainers seldom below par. The place enjoys a gambling concession, of which there are not very many, because the state prefers to have the profits flow through the Casino Nacional. As elsewhere, roulette seems to be the favorite game.

Sans Souci, the *Jockey Club*, *Mulgoba* and most of their popular rivals are suburban, too. The newest vogue is for sites on the highway leading to the Rancho Boyeros airport, which is natural enough. The old *Montmartre*, Calle P off Calle 23, Vedado, is considered downtown for a night club, and except for a few spots in famous hotels the clubs of the center, on and about the Prado, have lost their former standing. No type of business changes more rapidly. I hesitated over giving the names of any establishments, because they might have closed down before this book was printed. But I feel that those mentioned will endure.

Of small neighborhood resorts and ephemeral "dives" there is no end. A row of shacks on the main street leading to the beach at Miramar allured bohemians several years ago and came to be known as Las Fritas from the fried stuffs sold. The impromptu entertainment—rumbas and other country dances, popular ballads, guitar-playing—was genuinely Cuban. Though it is all more pretentious nowadays, it is not fatally so, and the bars of Las Fritas are worth a tour. One of the places that has had a long run is called the *Pennsylvania*; another is the *Panchín*.

With legal gambling available on every hand in Havana, notably at the Casino and the Jockey Club, it is strange that anybody should wish to practice the illegal kind. Yet many visitors do. They find forbidden spots easily enough, close to the Prado or in Chinatown. The latter is a relatively large district, west of Galiano and south of Zanja. As in other countries, the Chinese of Cuba cannot be induced to forego their special games of chance, which they are willing to share under certain conditions with thrill-seeking foreigners.

The male night-hawk is likely to want to round out his flitting with a look at the houses of prostitution, a rough generic term perhaps, for some of them are extremely elegant. At no time has the *fille de joie* been driven from Havana, or even seriously hampered in her calling, and there have been periods (see Chapters 10 and 15) when she reached fantastic heights of favor and prosperity. Under the republic sexual license is held to have been most extreme during the presidencies of Gómez, Zayas, and Machado, though it would be hard to prove that there was less of it when Grau was in power. At about the middle of the Prio administration a sudden spasm of reform (in this matter only, while graft was rampant) led to the closing of all the known houses and the jailing of free lances. The traffic was supposed to end, but nothing of the kind happened. The girls in the night bars were not touched, and before long harlots swarmed on the streets as they had been prevented from doing under the former system.

What had been accomplished was the vacating of hundreds of dwellings which were at once occupied by respectable tenants, persons who had not been able to find a place to live because of the housing shortage. The chief clean-up was of the Colón quarter, lying immediately west of the lower Prado. It satisfied an old complaint that the district was too valuable to be left to "red light" activities. The minister in charge of the reform, however, was touched with fanaticism which proved unpopular. He was dropped from the cabinet six months before Prío fell. Gradually the traffic was resumed, but in new locations and at greater distances from the center.

One of the houses on the Calle Colón may be said to have had world-wide celebrity. It was an ornate mansion from the past, of three stories and a patio decked with potted shrubs and palms. A tastefully furnished little bar had been built on the ground floor; it had space for a few couples to dance. Against this background moved girls in evening gowns, pretty, well-mannered girls who if anything seemed a little old-fashioned. There was never any drunkenness or loud talk. Men who rang the doorbell were not admitted unless known or obviously desirable. Connoisseurs came as to a club where the high prices were justified by the atmosphere. Though finished at that address, the house must be mentioned in any account of night life in modern Havana. The proprietress has reopened in the suburbs.

On the other hand, some very sordid and some very rowdy resorts existed in the suppressed tenderloin. They have been weeded out and should stay weeded. It would take a fresh mood of indifference and years of degeneration to produce the equal of the Calle Bernal as it was three years ago.

Chapter 39

NOT PASSED BY THE CENSOR

A POLICE CHIEF in the time of Menocal, loftily critical of his predecessor under José Miguel Gómez, is reputed to have suppressed the public showing of pornographic motion pictures with the comment that men who paid for sexual excitement should spend the money on living Cubans. Another official barred foreign prostitutes, remarking that the native-born were entitled to be protected from competition. Whether it is true or not that these words were uttered, the spirit of them prevails. Much *risqué* entertainment is offered in Havana, of local origin and in the flesh. Imported naughtiness really is frowned upon.

Let us ignore the outrageous exhibitions staged in the bordellos. They are lacking in imagination, and their like are to be seen in many countries. Anyone who pays the fancy prices charged is just a sucker. But here and there throughout the city you come upon variety shows which have a certain merit. They are all founded upon burlesque of the kind that was popular in New York before World War I, with Latin touches, and with the strip tease carried to ultimate conclusions. No doubt they go beyond the letter of the law, but the police wink at them so long as the audiences are composed almost entirely of Spanish-speaking males. Cuban women, of course, would not dream of attending. A scattering of tourists, even an occasional female tourist, is ignored. But if foreigners start coming in large numbers the place is closed, on the theory that it will give Havana a bad name abroad. It is pretty sure to reopen somewhere else.

On the edge of the Chinese quarter a theater of this sort has existed for a long time. I shall not name it, but identification by a visitor is not difficult since it advertises discreetly and every bartender and taxidriver knows about it. A typical program opens with a longish skit which an outsider will probably find boring, resting as it does upon dialect and local allusions. The short acts follow: some of them dramatized jokes, some song-and-dance, and others a species of bawdy pantomime. Hawkers improve the occasion by selling indecent booklets in the aisles.

You hear an appealing song now and then, or see a good dance number. Generally these phases of the entertainment are crude, with the emphasis on noise and gymnastics. The girl-appeal tableaux may be shameless, but they often have originality and at least they are silent; they constitute the most popular feature. Here is one that earned a grin from me:

The scene was a deserted city square at night, indicated by backdrops with street lamps painted in and the silhouettes of houses. There sauntered on stage a woman totally nude except for her hat and shoes, and swinging a handbag. Her implied calling was unmistakable. She produced a mirror from her bag and went through the motions of making up her face under a lamp. Presently she was joined by half a dozen sisters of the pavement, all in a similar state of undress. They talked by means of grimaces and shrugs which established the fact that business was poor indeed. Then appeared a tall and robust female, naked too except for a policeman's cap, brogans and a baton. The newcomer scowled at the harlots, menaced them with her nightstick, lined them up and proceeded to search them for concealed weapons. The comedy of this last operation was broad. I need say no more. Disgusted at having found nothing, the "cop" shooed her victims into the wings and strode off herself, while the orchestra struck up a quickstep.

The X Theater, however, is not the place for seeing art in undress—and there is such art. If you know where to look, you can find in some back street a small show revolving around a girl impassioned for success who dances nude as the only way of coming to the notice of managers. Occasionally, just occasionally, a girl of the sort puts money in second place. She is touched with genius which must find its outlet, and through her there emerges the fascinating truth that the dance was invented first and costumes afterward. Certain flowing lines are of the body and nothing else. Consequently there are measures which should be danced naked.

A room on a ground floor with a roughly built stage may serve as the theater, or it may even be a back yard with open-air seats and a canopied platform subdivided by curtains. The admission will scarcely be more than twenty-five cents. I recall a show in a setting of the kind. A swarthy girl, lithe and intense, was before the audience for the greater part of the hour that it lasted; the comedian with her was just a foil, though he headed the act. She danced six or seven times, in costume and out of it. The watchers applauded loudest when she was nude, and not for aesthetic reasons. But she did not seem to care one way or the other. Her black eyes were focused upon the moon.

Like most New World Chinatowns, the one in Havana has its morbidly secretive side, its dens where opium is smoked and other vices practiced. The visitor would do well to steer clear of them. Few guides would risk showing him the way, anyhow, and he would never find it for himself. If he cannot be satisfied unless he has had a glimpse at degradation, let him go no farther than some of the open bars on Zanja near San Nicolás, and down the side alleys. He will see marijuana addicts and drunkards. Cubans generally speaking are not inclined to alcoholism, but the wrecks in Chinatown who swallow crude liquor at five cents a glass are simply using the easiest and cheapest means of stunning their nerves.

Chapter 40

THE PAGEANT OF CARNIVAL

CARNIVAL IS one of Havana's great attractions toward the end of the winter season. The Tourist Commission does everything in its power to promote and publicize it. The effort is successful because it is a unique pageant, owing much to the Mardi Gras celebrations of New Orleans yet departing from them, and quite frankly overstepping the churchly origin of the festival. Carnival took form throughout the Roman Catholic world as an outburst of merriment on the eve of the rigors of Lent, and it stopped with the dawning of Ash Wednesday. But in Cuba it merely begins that week. There are parades and fiestas every Saturday and Sunday during Lent, up till Holy Week. It will be impossible to understand this without stepping backward into history.

The Church never favored Carnival; it tolerated it during periods when the people were difficult to control, and at other times it suppressed it. Pre-Lenten dances for the purpose of collecting funds for charity could hardly be forbidden, and those who took part adopted the custom of wearing masks. An early ordinance provided that a mask could be used only on the way to a ballroom, but this became a dead letter. The fun lay in mystifying one's friends—and one's enemies too. About the middle of the nineteenth century, children were given permission to be in the streets masked on Shrove Tuesday, and this privilege was soon extended to slaves. Adult citizens had to take it for themselves, and very often they misused it. The mask was a cover for acts of vengeance and law-breaking generally.

There were two sorts of parade, the first of more or less distinguished persons in carriages or on horseback; the second of associations known as *comparsas*, the members of which usually went afoot in extravagant disguises. The earliest parades of the genteel were along Carlos III, and the emulation consisted wholly in the brilliant costumes of the women, the liveries of the coachmen and grooms, and the escort of gallant cavaliers. The comparsas roamed over town at will. A great deal of jesting took place between the paraders and the crowds that lined the sidewalks. *Mamarrachos*, or carnival clowns, were recognized figures who under cover of their masks made mock of the authorities. More than one riot broke out as a result of the audacity of these fellows.

Spanish medieval beliefs inspired the first comparsas.

Their shows consisted of carrying the Virgin in procession with attendant saints and hunting down the Devil, usually portrayed as a serpent. But Negroes, both free and slaves, became tremendously attached to the notion of comparsas. They formed their own societies, which they called *cabildos*, and introduced details from African animistic faiths. The comparsas came to be regarded as typically Negro. The Day of the Kings (January 6) had been adopted by the blacks, and on that occasion they ran wild, dancing and miming, collecting tribute in cash from the amused spectators. The Negro acts seen later in Carnival had nearly all been created on the Day of the Kings.

In certain years under the Spaniards the colored people were forbidden to send out their comparsas, for fear that they might serve to cover an uprising of slaves. But in 1886, when slavery was abolished, the ban was lifted and not imposed again until the outbreak of the War of Independence. The republic allowed a revival in 1902.

Carnival as we know it today was shaped under the republic. In 1908 the first floats—*Gulliver's Travels, Scenes from the Middle Ages*, and others—were brought from New Orleans. That same year the first "Queen of the Carnival" was elected, a beauty who was married in La Merced church on the last Sunday of the season with officials and members of the diplomatic corps in attendance. Since then, Havana has managed the building of its own floats and has developed one of the most elaborate fiestas held anywhere in the world. A condensation of the official program for 1952 will give an idea of it.

The queen, chosen from a large number of competitors, was crowned in the Anfiteatro Nacional by the President of Cuba himself, on the evening of February 22nd, the Friday preceding Lent.

The following evening occurred the inaugural parade of

Carnival, with floats, led by the queen who was accompanied by maids of honor who had been runners-up to her in the contest, visiting beauties and damsels chosen for their pulchritude by Cuban organizations. The route was from the Parque de Maceo, by way of the Malecón and the Prado to the Plaza de la Fraternidad. Splendid costumes were seen. The chief reviewing stand was in front of the Capitol.

On Sunday the 24th there was an informal promenade, with decorated open automobiles and other vehicles, which took the long route from the Maine Monument to the Plaza de la Fraternidad.

After that, in opposition to the New Orleans custom, there were no program features until Lent had started. Even Mardi Gras Day, February 27th, passed without any important celebration.

Friday the 29th was the occasion of a fashion and flower show in the Centro Asturiano, presided over by the First Lady of the Republic.

March 1st saw the first of the four Saturday evening parades of the comparsas. The groups called themselves by such names as Marquesses and Sultanas, the Dandies of Belén, and the Gypsies. Drummers and players of *mambo* music accompanied them. They carried *farolas* ("transparencies") at the tops of long poles. After the third and fourth parades judges awarded prizes for local color, artistry, and stylized treatment.

The intervening Sundays were devoted to promenades similar to the one held on February 24th, but varied by exhibition bicycle-riding, popular Cuban dances, and folk songs. In the afternoon of the third Sunday there was also a series of historical tableaux staged in original settings as follows:

Plaza de la Catedral: A slaves' jamboree.

Plaza de Armas: A meeting of the old colonial municipal council.

La Fuerza Castle: Doña Isabel de Bobadilla and her ladies.

The Paula Church: Religious ceremony in the manner of old times, with music by the Coro ("Choir") Nacional.

Wall of the Arsenal: The Inn called the Golden Galleon.

Loma del Angel: A scene from *Cecilia Valdés*, Cuba's classic novel, by Cirilo Villaverde.

Convent of San Francisco, now the General Post Office: A concert.

Convent of Santa Clara, now the Ministry of Public Works: A concert.

San Lázaro Tower: An ambush by pirates.

A Pan-American fiesta occurred in the morning on the last Sunday of Carnival. The amphitheater was decorated with the flags of all the free countries of the hemisphere. Typical songs and dances were rendered. Finally the different phases of the celebration found their climax in an open-air dance on the esplanade in front of the Capitol, from ten P.M. to midnight.

The whole season is marked by private balls, generally in masquerade. One of the country clubs always gives a smart ball on Shrove Tuesday. The Centro Gallego, Centro Asturiano, and Centro de los Dependientes, located where the tides of Carnival flow strongest, put on huge affairs each week end. Dances for children are held by many of the clubs on Saturday afternoons; it is noteworthy that the participants are costumed like their elders and zealously imitate the latter as northern children would scarcely do.

Chapter 41

NANIGO, OR CUBAN HOCUS-POCUS

MANY REFERENCES have been made in these pages to
ñáñigo, the secret Negro cult that has always been a factor
in western Cuba (see Chapter 15). Visitors hear that the
more flamboyant comparsas in the carnival parades are from
"voodoo societies"—meaning ñáñigo. It is also bruited that
the old weird ceremonies are still performed and can be
seen if you are taken by the proper guide. A little truth lies
at the bottom of all this. Náñigo at its extremest employed
hocus-pocus rather than malignant witchcraft, and now it
is not so sensational as it used to be. It still sends out its
comparsas on the Day of the Kings and the Saturday eve-
nings of Carnival, and it has other ways of expressing itself.
Only an authority, such as the great Cuban folklorist Dr.
Fernando Ortiz, could define what ñáñigo really is. But it
is not voodoo.

An anonymous writer tells how on the Day of the Kings
in 1863 the Negroes, slaves as well as freemen, monopolized
the open spaces of the city as tradition allowed them to do.
The women wore vivid, extravagant costumes. There was
wild hilarity, leaping and dancing to the rhythm of long
African drums played by striking them with the palm of the
hand. At twelve noon, that year's king and queen of the
blacks called at the palace of the captains general, the pair

being a very old Negro man and a woman so fat that she needed two strong chairs to support her when she sat down. That they came as the delegates of the ñáñigo societies is not to be doubted. The governor received them ceremoniously, allowed their followers to enter the patio and dance, and then distributed presents. It was an acknowledgment of good will, the extension of a truce.

But in some years no such pleasant state of affairs prevailed. The various Negro groups would clash in bloody riots. There would be an outbreak of crime, attributed rightly or wrongly to the practitioners of ñáñigo. The cult would be ordered suppressed, an end that was never attained though a majority of the leaders were often rounded up and imprisoned. Negro participation in street masquerades would be banned for long periods. This seesaw of favor and disfavor continued under the republic. The last prohibition of the comparsas was lifted in 1935, and there does not seem much likelihood that it will ever again be applied.

Náñigo went its way, holding its secret lodge meetings and finding public contacts by associating itself with certain Catholic festivals. San Lázaro—the Lazarus of the New Testament, the "beggar full of sores"—has become in Cuba the saint of Negroes, as well as of paupers, prostitutes, the ill and the disinherited. Altars to him are set up on December 17th. Those in the Negro quarters of Havana, in Regla across the harbor, in Guanabacoa and other suburban points, are often startling mixtures of Christian and animistic symbolism. There will be a perfectly respectable figure of the saint, a crucifix, candles and flowers, but intermingled with these a bottle of rum, dishes filled with votive offerings of food, cornmeal strewn in an intricate maze, and little bunches of cocks' feathers.

If located in an interior room or a guarded patio, there will generally be musicians and dancing around the altar.

The constricted space is jammed tight with bodies of both sexes, twisting and swaying, jerking their heads from side to side, rotating their hips and lifting their palms in gestures of entreatment. That is how I saw it on one occasion. It has been said that devotion to San Lázaro among the whites is the most deeply rooted popular faith in Havana because of the yellow-fever pesthole that the city used to be. The chief hospital was named after him. Beguiled by the fervor, though little worried about diseases, the blacks adopted San Lázaro. On the feminine side, Santa Bárbara was their choice.

The Virgin of the Assumption, patroness of Guanabacoa, is the center of special rites on August 15th. Her image is paraded about the town. There follows, by custom, a great fiesta which appears to have nothing to do with religion. Negroes flock from Havana, Regla, and other points to take part in it. Wild balls used to be held by groups calling themselves the Mazukamba, the Baracuta and the Lloviznita. The first of these three names has survived. Theatrical display has lessened, but some strange and rowdy dances are still held in Guanabacoa on the night of the 15th.

Visitors are perfectly free to attend Negro places of worship on Saints' Days and the balls. If they bring the kind of eye that sees below surfaces, they should be able to distinguish where the element of ñáñigo comes in. But they will not find any ceremonies involving blood sacrifices, not even the blood of a white cock. If such exist they are conducted in the profoundest secrecy.

Chapter 42
BOOKS AND THE ARTS

HAVANA IS a city where large numbers of books are on sale at high prices, the few that are printed locally being relatively the most expensive. Even second-hand books are dear. The condition in a country otherwise so progressive is unfortunate. Cuba has no book publishers in the proper sense of the term. It has only printeries which will turn out a job for cash or on terms. The party taking the financial risk is too often the poor author himself. Costs are exorbitant because of the wage scale for printers and the price of materials. So it is common to be asked five dollars for a paper-covered volume, an almost prohibitive figure. Books imported from Mexico and Spain are cheaper. Those from the United States are marked up 10 per cent or more.

As in most Latin countries, the Government does a considerable amount of publishing, for the dissemination of patriotic ideas and the encouragement of literature. Thus, Cuba has offered prizes for the best biographies of José Martí and other leaders, has issued the works, and has also put out a handsome India-paper edition of the complete writings of Martí. National annals, assembled by the Academy of History and other agencies, are lavishly preserved in print by the state.

There is no modern Cuban novel of the stature of *Cecilia*

Valdés, none that catches the spirit of the period as Villa-verde's story caught that of the nineteenth century. The poets have shown greater vigor. Dulce María Loynaz has been hailed in Spain as the most gifted woman poet in the language among her contemporaries, while Nicolas Guillén has proved an innovator with his Afro-Caribbean school of verse. The young Carilda Oliver Labra is justly admired.

The following are the chief book stores conveniently located for travelers:

Bohemia, on Neptuno facing the Parque Central; and *Swan*, on Obispo. These carry books in English.

Moderna Poesía, on Obispo; *Cervantes*, on Obispo; and *Albela*, on Belascoain. Spanish and English.

Casa Belga, on O'Reilly, French and English.

Mediedo, on O'Reilly. South American publications.

Librería Martí, on O'Reilly; *Librería Temis*, on O'Reilly; *Librería Economica*, on O'Reilly; *Editorial Lex*, on Obispo; *Minerva*, on Bernaza; *Cervantes*, on Galiano. Books in Spanish.

Editorial Gonzáles Porto, on Obispo. Technical books in various languages.

Pictorial art and sculpture are on a solid basis in Cuba. Much is owed to the San Alejandro school, founded in 1818 and directed for its first sixty years by French, Italian, and Spanish classicists. Finally a Cuban, Miguel Melero, was appointed director. He opened the classes to women. A great influence was exerted by Leopoldo Romañach, who died in 1951 when he was almost ninety, the acknowledged master of Cuban painting. Other names have been mentioned in the chapters on the National Museum and the Presidential Palace, which contain examples of their work. Among the good contemporary painters are Esteban Valderrama, Gerardo Tejedor, Manuel Mesa and the versatile Armando Maribona who is also a professor at San Alejandro, an author, and an active journalist on the staff of the *Diario de la Marina*. Some of the quite young are promising, but none is so outstanding that he can be appraised without question.

Native Cuban sculpture begins with José de Vilalta Saavedra, who died early in the present century, and culminates so far with the talented Juan José Sicre. The work of these two and of most others of importance figure in the chapter on Havana's monuments. It should also be noted that Mario Santí, who is both painter and sculptor, won the honor of building the pantheon in Santa Ifigenia Cemetery, Santiago de Cuba, to which the bones of José Martí have just been removed.

Several professional societies are most active in forwarding the interests of art. To cite the three most important according to age, there are the Asociación de Pintores y Escultores, the Club Cubano de Bellas Artes, and the Círculo de Bellas Artes. All have held many exhibitions. The Círculo, youngest of the three, has rooms on Industria immediately behind the Capitol, where any visitor is welcomed informally to practically continuous shows of the members' work. The Ministry of Education has held five national salons at irregular intervals. Important exhibitions have been sponsored by the municipality, the University of Havana, and by many cultural associations. An influential group which includes Armando Maribona is organizing a permanent gallery, where native painting and sculpture can be sold as well as seen, and through which exchange shows with foreign countries can be arranged.

Havana is a music-loving city. The Sociedad Pro Arte Musical, founded in 1918, which built the Auditorium in the Vedado (see Chapter 37), has given and still gives a tremendous stimulus to the presenting of good programs. It has brought famous symphony orchestras and the most celebrated artists from Europe, and at the same time has neglected no opportunity to put forward real Cuban talent. The Sociedad Coral de la Habana (choral music) and the Orquesta de Cámera (chamber music) are both extremely active. The Lyceum y Lawn-Tennis Club, though a general cultural organization for women, traditionally devotes the major share of its indoor activities to music.

Cuban composers who developed native themes have been numerous, from the mulatto José Silvestre White who died at eighty-two in 1918, to Ernesto Lecuona, a modern whose work is well-known in the United States.

The dance enjoys an ardent following. In Alicia Alonso, a young contemporary, Havana has produced a ballet star of international reputation. She often appears with her company at the Auditorium. Fine exponents of the Spanish dance, flamenco as well as classical, never lack public support. Then we have the wide range of local measures, which are interpreted well or ill in the night clubs and cabarets. The average tourist knows about the rumba and the more recent *mambo*, and with them his information ceases. Ten to one, he believes them to be numbers which would be acceptable in polite drawing rooms.

But the rumba (often spelled rhumba in English, without rhyme or reason) is strictly an exhibition dance, a pantomime of sex desire and mating, which originated among plantation Negroes in slavery times. The man pursues and the woman gradually yields to persuasion. He struts like a barnyard cock when it is clear that his point has been gained, and she flees from the stage on a note of bawdy comedy. The tempo throughout is very rapid. The ruffles on the costumes are supposed to represent fowl's feathers. It used to be considered that an ideal team was a robust, plump mulatto woman and a small black man. The handsomest young couples render it now.

The mambo has been described as a frenziedly jazzed

version of the *danzón*, a graceful old Cuban measure.
Danzón, *danza* and *son* all had the same characteristics:
they were done to slow music, which quickened at intervals and then would mark time enabling the couples to
stop dead and talk in whispers before a fresh quirk of the
orchestra started them going again. It is said that the
pauses of the danzón provided the only opportunity that
well-bred young persons had for flirting at a ball. Romantic
dignity of that sort has been swept away by the mambo.
The older generation disapproves, but can do nothing about
it, except to insist that the mambo, like the rumba, must
be confined to the cabarets.

Chapter 43

CIGARS, PERFUMES AND SO FORTH

TOBACCO as an industry holds second place, immediately after sugar though far behind it, in the economy of
Cuba. Many of the great cigar and cigarette factories are
in Havana. Travelers always have found them worth visiting, and the management extends a welcome. Cigarettes,
to be sure, are made by machinery nowadays, and there is
little interest in watching the process. But the best cigars
are still rolled by hand, and the technique is fascinating.
Though cigar machines have been invented, it is claimed
that a perfect job can be done only by a human operator.

An expert can roll about two hundred cigars a day. To abolish artists of the sort would be a crime against skilled labor.

The Tabacalera Cubana, one of the largest companies, maintains a museum at Zulueta 106, opposite the Presidential Palace. Here are shown a carved group of Siboney Indians in front of their thatched hut, inhaling through forked tubes the smoke of burning tobacco; various paintings illustrating the development of the trade with Europe; wall-cases with exhibits of the leaf in all its stages, tools, and soils; and other novelties. The fact is emphasized that Columbus first observed the use of tobacco in Cuba.

Four clever operators, two women and two men, are continuously at work behind a railing. The women are strippers, eliminating the ribs of the leaves without tearing the filler. The men twist the last-named in the proper way, cover it with wrapper, and mold and trim the whole into a cigar with incredible speed. The color of the wrapper fixes the general type of the brand, ranging from *claro* (light) to *maduro* (very dark), though the quality is of course determined by the filler. A pale tinge does not prove that a cigar is mild, any more than a dark wrapper insures strength. The tradition exists, however, and filler and wrapper are combined accordingly.

The demonstrators in the museum are representative of scores of workers in large rooms upstairs. By ancient custom they are entertained while on the job by a professional reader who sits on a raised platform and gives them scenes from fiction or drama. The newly made cigars are dried for a few days in special cabinets, and are then packed in the regulation boxes which if not wholly of cedar must be lined with that wood to keep the tobacco in good condition.

Fine Havana cigars are far from cheap. They never have been. The latest is a long, fat smoke called a Churchill, which retails at one dollar, a fancy price even in Cuba. The story goes that it was created for the British Prime Minister when he last visited Havana, that 500 were presented to him as a parting gift and his blessing upon the name secured. The average twenty-five cent Havana can be rated as excellent.

Cubans smoke far more cigars per capita than North Americans do, and they also use great numbers of the strong local cigarettes, which retail at an average price of ten cents for a package of sixteen. The industry, comprising exports and home consumption, goes beyond a value of $100,000,000 in most years.

Much smaller, but on a sound basis and with possibilities for the future, is the manufacture of perfumes and cosmetics. It is mainly a Havana business, some of the firms being entirely Cuban while others are branches of famous European companies. Tourists buy more and more of the product, because of the attractive prices. In the case of certain brands which directly compete with perfumes made in the United States, travelers may take back with them only one bottle free of duty. Otherwise the full limit of the customs exemption may be applied to such purchases.

Largest of the Cuban firms is Crusallas y Cía. Its liveliest competitor and the one that most hospitably encourages inspection is the Perfumería Fibah, established on the Chateau Madrid estate, Marianao, just outside Havana. The name Fibah derives from *Habif*, spelled backward. The Habif family came from Turkey not so many years ago and founded the French Doll, a successful downtown shop for tourists. There followed other ventures, culminating in this perfume manufactury. Mauricio Habif showed me how the processes are applied. The concentrated essences are imported from France, he said, for tropical

flowers are comparatively weak in odor and as yet no outstanding variations have been created from them. The
scents of leaves and grasses are more promising, and a new
one for which much is hoped is about to be launched.

As a show place the Chateau Madrid surpasses anything
of the kind in Havana. On its fourteen landscaped acres
are gardens and experimental farms, birds and monkeys in
cages, peacocks roving free, a fishpond, a cottage amid the
branches of a huge guinep (*mamoncillo*) tree. There is a
restaurant for the staff and favored guests, and a gift shop
in which the range is from good jewelry to souvenirs cheaply
priced. As many as 1,100 visitors have appeared at the
Chateau Madrid in a single day, most of them tourists.
Yet Habif smilingly observes that entertaining tourists is
merely a form of promotion which his company believes
will create good will. The reliance is upon the shops of
Cuba, which buy the greater part of the luxury goods he
produces, and retailers from Cuban country towns form an
important percentage of those who come to call.

The Perfumería Fibah makes lotions, colognes and soaps
as well as perfumes, and it will soon be turning out cosmetics of all sorts.

Another product which interests the shopper from abroad
is alligator leather. The West Indian reptile from which
it is obtained is really a crocodile, but the scientific distinction is ignored and alligator remains the popular term.
Cuba has a huge supply of the creatures, especially in the
Zapata marsh on the south coast, and the manufacture of
ladies' handbags, shoes, belts, and other articles from the
hides has become an important Havana industry. Prices are
considerably lower than they would be in the United States.

Mahogany items, fans, and tiles compete with alligator-
leather goods in the souvenir shops. Cigarette and other
boxes, candy and nut platters, bookends, etc., are made

from the king of tropical woods. The best fans are imported from Spain or the Orient, though some of the cheap local designs are not at all bad. There has long been a Cuban industry in tiles, used for paving floors, corridors and patios, and as a facing for walls. Enthusiasts collect them and hang the more striking in lieu of pictures.

Rum, of course, has top-rank appeal. The larger distilleries are all in the provinces. The Bacardí Company and the Havana Rum Company maintain city headquarters where, as I have told, the traveler is genially received. It should be noted that some of the best Cuban brands are made in accordance with a brandy formula and so do not resemble the heavy Jamaica-type liquor which the average outsider associates with the word rum. There are some good Cuban cordials, especially those of pineapple and banana flavors.

Chapter 44

FAMOUS RESTAURANTS AND BARS

FEW CITIES in the Western Hemisphere equal Havana in the matter of agreeable restaurants that serve good food. The best comparison is with New Orleans in the latter's palmy days. Both have developed a special Creole cuisine, the one based upon Spanish and the other upon French. Both are famous for their seafood. The following is a representative list of eating places, including those that are well known and some obscure places which I have found excellent.

La Zaragozana, on Monserrate opposite the Centro Asturiano. This is the oldest high-class restaurant in Havana. It was founded in 1830 and there is some resemblance to the celebrated Antoine's, of New Orleans, founded ten years later. Calmly old-fashioned, La Zaragozana maintains its standards in the face of modern competition, charges high prices and is approved by Cubans and foreigners alike. It specializes in fish and shellfish dishes. Better Moro crab, natural or stuffed, is not to be found anywhere. And the menu is large and varied, the wine list impressive.

Restaurant Paris, in the ancient palace of the Marquisses de Aguas Claras sometimes called the Ponce de León palace, on the Plaza de la Catedral. I bracket the Paris with the Zaragozana because they are probably the two most distinguished eating places. The Paris, however, is less Cuban. It features an international cuisine, and its French wines are of the best. The setting of the Paris is superior, for in addition to the noble architecture of the patio there is a terrace on the plaza which commands a view of the cathedral. When there is moonlight and guitarists come to play soft melodies, as they did in colonial times, the effect is magical.

La Florida, at Obispo and Monserrate. One of the really fine places. Game, poultry and shellfish are specialties.

Ambos Mundos, at Obispo and Mercaderes. There are two restaurants run by the hotel of that name, one on its roof (see Chapter 31) and one on the ground floor of a building opposite. The roof is preferred by visitors, but Havana connoiseurs value the culinary merits of the less spectacular restaurant.

Armando's, on the ground floor of the Hotel Inglaterra,

facing the Parque Central. Harmoniously decorated with colored tiles. Very Cuban in character, and the food moderately priced.

Miami, at Prado and Neptuno. By no means a tourist trap, as its name would seem to imply. A first-line Havana eating house, offering an elaborate menu. The fruit salads are particularly good.

Cosmopolita-El Patio, on the lower Prado. Two established names have combined in a picturesque house that stands back amid shrubbery and flowers. Formerly it was just El Patio.

El Palacio de Cristal, at Consulado and San José, with a side view of the Capitol. North Americans often overlook this dignified place which used to be extremely exclusive, with its rows of private alcoves (*reservados*) entered from Consulado. Its spacious main dining room is now much patronized for banquets by organizations. An all-around menu, but the best dishes should be ordered well in advance.

Prado 86, on the lower Prado. Called after the original street number before a new system made it in fact Prado Number 264. Formerly a club.

El Templete, on the Avenida del Puerto. Most of the seating is at open-air sidewalk tables. Specializes in all kinds of seafood.

El Toledo, at Aguila and Barcelona. Decorated in a garish Spanish style. Good surprises on the menu.

La Reguladora, Amistad between Barcelona and Dragones. A favorite luncheon place for businessmen of the neighborhood.

El Ariete, at San Miguel and Consulado. A small, intimate place, with reservados, that keeps very late hours.

La Pescadora, at Cárcel 55, a survivor in an old neighborhood that has largely been swept away by reconstruction for the landscaping of the waterfront.

La Bodeguita del Medio, on Empedrado near the cathedral. A truly bohemian spot. The restaurant grew spontaneously in the back-room and then the yard of a small grocery shop. It is crowded at lunchtime by neighborhood patrons, but in the evening is frequented by writers and practitioners of all the arts.

La Maravilla, on the Plaza del Cristo. A *fonda*, or small Hispanic eating house, with a reputation for steaks. It has long been a favorite of mine.

Club Palermo, at San Miguel and Amistad. Comparatively new, it combines the attractions of good food and night-club music.

La Isla, at Galiano and San Rafael, with back entrances to reservados on Rayo. First-class Cuban and Spanish food. The catering is typical of older days in Havana.

Del Pacífico, on San Nicolás near Zanja. This is a genuine Chinese restaurant located on the rooftop of a Chinatown hotel, and it does not compromise with western tastes.

La Sevilla, the restaurant of the Sevilla-Biltmore Hotel, on the Prado. Very good along international lines, as is to be expected in hotels of this grade.

La Arboleda, the main restaurant of the Hotel Nacional, O and 21, Vedado. What was said in the preceding paragraph applies equally to La Arboleda and to *Chez Merito*, the restaurant of the Hotel Presidente, on the Avenida de los Presidentes at Calzada, Vedado.

Hotel Vedado, at 19 and M, Vedado. Offers a good table d'hôte meal, with Cuban dishes featured.

El Carmelo, with two branches in the Vedado, the chief establishment being at Calzada and D, and the lesser one at 23 near the Avenida de los Presidentes. Enjoys a vogue, but seems imitation Californian rather than Cuban to me.

La Concha, at the beach of the same name, Marianao. The fruit salad is special, but there are many good things on the menu. You eat at outdoor tables shaded by palm-leaf parasols.

Rio Cristal, on the road to Rancho Boyeros airport. Of the many restaurants in the outskirts, I choose this one for mention because of the great charm of its setting. The building was once a convent. The gardens are beautifully laid out, and there is plenty of running water with a swimming pool. In order to keep out undesirables, Rio Cristal is organized as a club.

Most Havana eating places have bars, but it is not usual for the bar to have a clientele apart from the restaurant. *La Florida*, often called *La Floridita*, is an exception. This bar is famous for its Daiquirí cocktails, which many drinkers aver to be the best in the city. The bar of *Ambos Mundos*, across the way from the front door of the hotel, also is patronized on its own account.

Sloppy Joe's, at Zulueta and Animas, must be mentioned because it is undoubtedly the bar best known to the general run of tourists. The name was publicized during the prohibition era, when certain North Americans came to Havana with the sole idea of drinking and rather liked the implication that they could be as sloppy as they pleased. Joe accommodated bibulous women with belts of miniature bottles to be worn under their skirts and smuggled into the United States. It was a stupid, noisy resort, and now it is utterly commonplace.

The institution of the night bar has been dealt with elsewhere (see Chapter 38). Probably *Johnny's Bar Club*, on Virtudes off the Prado, is the best-known of this type. The bar of the Plaza Hotel falls into the category. So, with diminishing decorum, do a number of bars close to the waterfront of Old Havana.

This is as good a spot as any to mention that absinthe, barred in most countries because of a slight drug content which the moralists say is habit-forming, is legal in Cuba. You may order absinthe drip or absinthe frappée in any bar, but it is strictly forbidden to take back even one drop to the United States.

Chapter 45

TYPICAL CUBAN DISHES

ASK THE newly arrived visitor what food he associates in his mind with Cuba, and he will probably name *arroz con pollo*. But this is a very simple dish, eaten in every Spanish country. It means "rice with chicken," and while it is seasoned in a variety of ways the basic ingredients are chicken and rice yellowed with saffron, steamed together. The original of all such dishes is the *paella* of Spain, sometimes made with meat, sometimes with fish and shellfish. Here is a typical recipe employed in Havana.

Paëlla Valenciana
Half a cup of olive oil
One chicken
Half a pound of bacon
Half a pound of ham
One pimiento, chopped up

One tomato, chopped up
Garlic, salt and pepper
Annatto paste (reddish)
One large cup of rice

Wait until the olive oil has been well heated in a casserole. Add the bacon, the ham and the chicken, cut up
into small pieces. When the meat is browning well, add
the pimiento and the tomato, with enough water to cover
everything. Add black pepper ground fine, with other
flavorings and enough annatto paste to give the color desired. After the contents of the casserole has simmered for
a while, put in the rice. Add enough broth or water to
cook the rice without burning it. Once the rice has started
to cook, do not add any more water. When fully cooked,
shake down the casserole and leave on the stove as long as
needed for the excess liquid to evaporate.

The above recipe will undoubtedly be too oily to suit
all tastes. The bacon can be left out and more tomatoes
used.

Cangrejo Moro (Moro crab), a name that has nothing
to do with Morro Castle, as some tourists imagine. Moro
means "Moorish." This is a variety of stone crab with very
large black-tipped claws. If ordered *natural*, the claw-meat
only is served cold, with mayonnaise. But the masterpiece
is stuffed Moro crab, the titbits of several crustaceans being
used to pack one of the large shells and the result baked.
Different restaurants treat in different ways, the least imagi-
native of which is *au gratin*.

Langosta (rock lobster), really a giant crawfish. The
body is thick with meat down to the tail, but the claws
are insignificant. Delicious broiled with a spiced sauce, or
cold with mayonnaise. The small freshwater crawfish are
called *langostinos* (little lobsters) and shrimps *camarones*.

Both are excellent and appear in many recipes. *Ostiones* (Cuban oysters) are tiny, but savory.

Pargo (red snapper, also called in English mutton-fish). The variety found in Cuban waters is the best of all the local fish. The flesh is firm and white, and of a delicate flavor. Pargo appears on virtually all menus in Havana, cooked in every conceivable manner. You cannot go wrong ordering it. One of the best styles is *almendrina*, which means a covering of crushed almonds with a butter sauce.

Other popular fish are *serrucho* (kingfish), *aguja* (sailfish), *atun* (tuna), *pámpano* (pompano), and all the small, succulent species known in southern Florida. If you want a mixed seafood grill, order *rancho de mariscos*.

Ajiaco. This is the down-to-earth native thick soup, a large helping of which is a meal. All the tropical vegetables are used—plantain, yam, taro, sweet potato, yuca (cassava), tomato, green pepper, onion, and corn-on-the-cob sliced into counters—and pork as the basic enrichment. The ajiaco of a poor country family may contain no meat except scraps of crackling. In a good city restaurant there will be salt pork and pieces of smoked ham.

Many soups of European origin are eaten. For instance, *olla podrida*, which is the Spanish version of pepper pot; *fabada asturiano*, which utilizes every kind of bean, with a pork base; *caldo gallego*, made with white beans, potatoes and herbs, flavored with a little chicken and ham; *potaje de garbanzos*, a foundation of chick peas, with other vegetables and spiced sausage; and *sopa de cebolla*, which is French onion soup.

Congrí (rice and black beans) is often listed as a soup, though more resembling an hors d'oeuvre. The rice and beans are cooked separately and then mixed with chopped onion, oil, and vinegar. A very Cuban dish.

Picadillo (beef hash). This is not so commonplace an

item as the name might suggest. The local hash is deliciously seasoned, and some of the leading restaurants modify it in their own way. Usually served with a fried egg and rice.

Tamale (Cuba's version of a famous Mexican dish). It is made with grated fresh corn, with chicken or pork mixed in, onion and a spicy tomato sauce.

Lechón (suckling pig). This is the favorite pork in all parts of the island. It is particularly associated with the Christmas and New Year holidays, taking the place that roast turkey holds in northern lands. In addition to its role in every household, suckling pig is peddled on the streets all through Christmas Week.

Huevos (eggs) and *tortillas* (omelettes). The customers in Havana are very fond of egg dishes. Some of the favorites are *pisto manchego*: scrambled eggs mixed with ham, shrimp, peas, tomato sauce, and asparagus; *huevos a la malagueña*, practically the same as the preceding, but cooked and served seething in a casserole; and *huevos al nido*, shirred eggs with chicken livers, truffles, and mushrooms, served with a wine sauce in a nest of potatoes Julienne. There is no end to the varieties of omelettes, even to a sweetish one made with fried ripe plantains.

Chapter 46

CUBAN FRUITS AND FRUIT DRINKS

TROPICAL FRUITS, as exemplified in Cuba, are worth special attention. Nowhere else are they so widely used in their natural state, for the flavoring of ices, and as *refrescos* (refreshments) which the people of the island sagely prefer to alcoholic drinks. Every fruit, the pulp of the sugar cane and many nuts are converted into beverages by one process or another. Lists have been published in books and magazine articles, but I have yet to find a complete one, and the translations of the Spanish names often have been incorrect. I shall endeavor to come close to filling that lack.

1: *Piña* (pineapple). This is the number one fruit of the West Indies for the double reason of general popularity, and the fact that it was rated chief among the indigenous fruits discovered by Columbus and his men. It is crushed and used as a drink in two ways. Either the juice is strained from the pulp, in which case it is called *piña colada*; or it is served unstrained and topped with a little shaved ice, as *piña sin colar*.

2: *Guanábana* (sour-sop). Indigenous. Large and irregularly shaped. Drinks made from this fruit rank second only in popularity to pineapple. Whipped with milk, sugar and ice, it is called a *champola de guanábana*; with water

254

and sugar a *guanábana con agua*. The flavor is unique and almost indescribable, something like a peach kernel mingled with very ripe banana pulp.

3: *Anón* (sweet-sop). Indigenous. Not unlike the guanábana, but a much smaller fruit, sweeter and without the other's curious tang. Better eaten in the original state. Drinks are made from it, however, either with or without milk.

4: *Chirimoya* (custard apple). Indigenous. Rich, creamy pulp which should be eaten raw. The flavor does not survive strongly in a drink.

5: *Mamey* (Cuban mammee). Indigenous. A sacred fruit to the aborigines of the Greater Antilles. Only men were allowed to eat it. The flesh is coarse, fibrous and reddish, the flavor peculiar. Cubans like it as a refresco, in ices, and plain.

6: *Caimito* (star apple). Indigenous. It gets its English name from the fact that when bisected the arrangement of the seeds embedded in pulp is starlike. A mild, subtle flavor, which is improved by mixing it with fresh orange.

7: *Zapote* (naseberry). This is the name used in Havana. In eastern Cuba it is called the *níspero*. Indigenous. It has a slightly granular pulp, sweet and seductively flavored. A great favorite with the aborigines.

8: *Guayaba* (guava). Indigenous. A small, round fruit, with pink pulp in some varieties and yellow in others. It is eaten raw by children, but is best for making preserves and jellies.

9: *Fruta Bomba* (papaya). Only in Havana, where *papaya* has a vulgar connotation, is this fruit called fruta bomba. In eastern Cuba the name is papaya, as in English. It has digestive properties and makes an ideal breakfast melon. Whirled in an electric mixer with crushed ice, the pulp emerges as a drink.

10: *Sandía* (watermelon). This and other melons are also reduced to a drinkable consistency by whirling in an electric mixer. The result is surprisingly good.

11: *Naranja* (orange). All the citrus fruits were introduced from Europe to the West Indies shortly after the discovery by Columbus. Methods of using the orange and preparing orange juice need scarcely be described.

12: *Toronja* (grapefruit). As familiar to travelers as the orange. The variety popular in Cuba, however, has a milder taste than the one commonly eaten in the United States.

13: *Limón* (lemon). Used for making standard lemonade, and the flavoring of ices and whiskey drinks.

14: *Lima* (lime). Used for making limeade, and the flavoring of ices and rum drinks.

15: *Tamarindo* (tamarind). The sticky, acid pulp which clings to seeds in a beanlike pod, makes a drink of exceptional merit for the quenching of thirst. Tamarind sweetmeats are popular also.

16: *Granada* (pomegranate). A slightly astringent but pleasant beverage is made from the rosy pulp that encloses the seeds.

17: *Granadilla* (passion flower fruit, or granadilla). Grows on a vine. The flesh is glutinous. Much used by Cubans for making beverages and desserts.

18: *Mango* (mango). There are many varieties, originally introduced from the Orient. Perhaps the favorite in Cuba is the *filipina*. The peachlike pulp is crushed to make a beverage, as well as preserves and pastes. Green mangoes stewed whole are delicious.

19: *Marañon* (cashew). Distantly related to the mango, but of a singular structure. The fleshy edible pulp is in reality a swollen stem from which hangs a kidney-shaped seed. This pulp is somewhat acid and can be eaten when dead ripe; it is used mostly for preserves. The seed is the familiar cashew nut.

20: *Plátano* (plantain). A large, coarse variety of the banana family that can only be eaten cooked.

21: *Platanillo* or *Platanito* (banana). These names mean "little" *plátano*. One seldom hears the word banana in Havana. There are many varieties. The one favored by Cuban taste is a small, sweet, yellow banana dubbed *Chino* (Chinese). The pulp is beaten up with milk in an electric mixer to make a heavy, sweetish drink.

22: *Uva* (grape). Standard grape juice from ripe grapes is prepared in the better places, and naturally is superior to the bottled product. I prefer the rare grape verjuice, a semi-transparent, greenish beverage made from the juice of unripe grapes and retaining a light and scented acidity. Crystals of fruit sugar are suspended in this verjuice, and they give the illusion of at once fermenting when swallowed.

23: *Higo* (fig). There are several local varieties of figs, and they are eaten raw, stewed, preserved in syrup and utilized in every other possible way.

24: *Tuna* or *Higo Chumba* (prickly pear). The fruit of a species of cactus. Good raw, or in preserves.

25: *Pomarosa* (rose apple). A wild fruit in which children delight. The flesh has a faint savor of rose petals.

26: *Mamoncillo* (guinep). Resembles a tart plum. The yellowish pulp about a single seed pops out readily when the green skin is broken. The fruit grows in abundant clusters on a tall tree.

27: *Aguacate* (avocado pear). This is the only tropical fruit from which the Cubans do not, to my knowledge, extract a beverage. It enjoys high favor, of course, as a salad because of its rich, oily flesh.

28: *Coco* (coconut). A universal standby. The water

of the green coconut is drunk as a beverage, which incidentally blends well with rum. The nut, when young and gelatinous, is eaten as a delicacy; when mature, it is ground and milk is pressed from it. Coconut goes into ices, candies, and preserves of every description.

29: *Almendra* (almond). Little known to outsiders, but superior to coconut milk, is the luscious drink pressed from crushed almonds. Pastes and candies are also manufactured from this nut.

30: *Caña* (sugar cane). Stalks of fresh sugar cane are crushed between rollers, and the greenish juice extracted is called *guarapo*. It is not so sweet as one might expect and makes a novel drink.

Chapter 47

SHOPPING IN HAVANA

ENOUGH has been said in previous chapters about important Cuban products to indicate what most travelers will want to buy. However, a few words about shopping in general may be helpful. Native rum is good, but it should not be overlooked that foreign wines, brandies, whiskeys, gins, and cordials are cheaper here than in the United States. French and Spanish perfumes are sold at attractive prices, and of course they are more famous than the local products. Only in the matter of cigars is the Cuban trademark supreme and unchallenged. Articles acquired as souvenirs are something else again; unless they are native they do not have a value of association. Many such are offered in Havana.

Apart from saying that El Encanto on Galiano is one of the best department stores in the world and that virtually anything can be bought there, I do not intend to give the names of shops and dealers. Vogues fluctuate, and small establishments come and go. It will be preferable to indicate the neighborhoods, in some cases the streets, where different needs can be satisfied.

The lower Prado as a whole is no longer exclusive. There are some very fine shops on it, including the branches of certain European firms, notably perfumers. At the end where it joins the Parque Central, spreading around the latter and on the ground floor of the Manzana de Gómez we find a type of general store which emphasizes the appeal to tourists in search of bargains. Tense competition among these places exists, with the result that they cut the margin of profit and offer some really good buys.

On Obispo in Old Havana and San Rafael in New, both of them at right angles to the Parque Central, are shops of a higher standard, mixed with some that are not so wonderful. San Rafael is now the street of the best shops, offering jewelry, porcelain objects, and elegant knick-knacks of all kinds. Neptuno running parallel with it has places of the same type, but is more general in its appeal. Obispo was once the superior, the mother, of San Rafael. Now it, along with O'Reilly that buttresses it, must take second place, with the single exception that they have the best book shops in Havana, San Rafael none, and Neptuno only a few. Monserrate has overflow shops, some of them second-hand and not particularly aimed at the visitor. Monte, crossing the far upper end of the Prado, is wholly

Cuban, even to its Woolworth Ten Cent store which is staffed by girls who do not speak a word of English.

For antique shops, look on Consulado and other streets in the immediate vicinity of the Parque Central.

When you reach Galiano in New Havana, you have come to an all-around shopping street, as North Americans understand the term. Here is El Encanto, at the corner of San Miguel; here another Woolworth's, along with a multiplicity of lesser rivals, of gift bazaars and groceries, interspersed with branches of almost all the foreign banks in Havana.

Belascoain, Infanta and other main crosstown arteries are centers of the retail trade, as is Calle 23 (sometimes called the Rampa) in the Vedado. But you will come back to Galiano as the one that is most satisfying. Oddly, the end nearest to the sea is just a jumble of residences, while the opposite extremity impinges upon Chinatown with a large public market on the northern side. This institution, known as the Vapor, has become the most important in central Havana since the Colón market behind the Presidential Palace was closed, to be reconstructed as a museum and gallery of fine arts. There is also the Unico, largest of all, at the Quatro Caminos (Four Roads) crossing near Atarés Castle.

You should not ignore these markets, though they offer few things that the tourist will want to buy. They are extremely picturesque, and for a certain sort of browser they hold rewards. He will see everything that he could possibly expect in a market, as well as a number of surprises. Loaded counters of fruits and vegetables, it goes without saying, more than it would seem possible to sell, in view of the competition outside. Meat, poultry, and fish stalls at which if you have a squeamish stomach it would be well not to look too closely. Dairy, grocery, candy, flower, basket, hardware, woodwork, and leather-goods shops. A shop for the sale of songbirds. And in addition to all these, a retail liquor store, tiny bars, restaurants, coffee stalls, fruit-juice stands, a billiard parlor; booths for secondhand articles of every description, and a shop where images of the saints, crucifixes and other objects of piety are offered. At the Unico I have even observed discarded grillwork from old houses in a formidable tangled heap.

The medley of odors in the markets is agreeable, except in the vicinity of the meat and the fish. Stallholders are wont to set out rows of vases containing vivid flowers. The market is loud with the singing of caged birds, not all of which are for sale. You cannot help noticing the large number of cats, the adults dozing on the counters among the goods, the kittens dashing about or perhaps curled in baskets and bowls. A first thought that Cubans are great lovers of cats has to be revised, for the evidence elsewhere in the city proves clearly that they are not. They make much of dogs and treat cats with indifference. But in the ancient markets they need some protection against the rats. There are men who seldom budge from these precincts. They live cheaply, for late at night I have seen sandwiches made from meat that would have spoiled by the next day being sold at very low prices.

A well-known oddity of Havana shopkeepers is not to use their own names, but to adopt some philosophical, poetical, or otherwise high-flown label. Thus, El Encanto (Enchantment) is what the noted department store calls itself. La Poesía Moderna (Modern Poetry) is a stationery and book store that does not pay special attention to poetry. El Pensamiento (Thought) is a dry-cleaning establishment, and another of the same name is a general clothing and linen store. La Purísima Concepción (The Immaculate Conception) is a grocery and bakery.

Chapter 48

THE TOURIST COMMISSION

ACTIVE and intelligent efforts are made to encourage tourism in Cuba. This is not to be wondered at, for after sugar it is the country's second or third largest moneymaker, according to the way you calculate. Tobacco is the challenger for second place, and if you include the value of the domestic consumption of tobacco it has the lead. But all the money spent by tourists—an average annually of $50,000,000—is an addition to the island's wealth. So Cuba has passed a law for the protection, even the coddling, of the tourist, with a special branch of the police to enforce it. Atop sits the Tourist Commission to originate new attractions and to help visitors in ways great or small.

La Corporación Nacional de Turismo, to use its official title for once, is a bureau of the Government of Cuba. Its president and commissioners are distinguished men, but these are apt to be replaced when a change in the national administration occurs. The permanent director of the office, which is at Cárcel 109, between the Prado and Morro, is Señor Miguel Santiago Valencia. A man of letters, a former journalist who spent many years in Paris, Valencia is in the right spot for the exercise of his talents. He is friendly, suave, and he speaks both English and French fluently.

The commission gets out a short guidebook, which is

revised each year; it prepares pamphlets, folders and maps, lists of recommended hotels, and mimeographed sheets giving miscellaneous information. All its publications are distributed free. It will answer any legitimate inquiry made by a traveler, draw up itineraries for excursions, obtain without charge a temporary permit for a visitor to drive a car. It will give the legal rate that taxis, porters and guides may charge. If any dispute arises, you may telephone the commission, which will send someone to handle the matter. Should court action follow, the stranger need not even make a personal appearance, for he will be represented by a delegate of the commission.

Such profuse service stems from the law referred to, which makes the tourist a favored individual. He may become drunk and noisy, he may commit any small offense, and the regular police will not touch him. They will steer him into the hands of the tourist police, whose members wear an arm-badge and who speak English. These specials will take him, if necessary, to their station house, sober him up and guide him to his hotel without having made a charge against him. On the positive side, he will be helped in an argument or fight by a tourist policeman, who generally will give the short end to the Cuban involved. The theory is, that the visitor is not familiar with local difficulties, and so should be treated as a guest and excused.

A major crime would of course land even a tourist in jail, but nothing short of that. There was the case of the playgirl "Satira" a few years ago who was convicted of murder on a yacht and sentenced to a long term in Príncipe Castle. But as her victim had been a countryman of her own, the sentence was soon commuted to deportation. Luckily for her, reparation for the life of a Cuban had not imposed itself.

The tourist corps of the police was created as the result

of recommendations by the Tourist Commission. The latter holds the authority to license all guides, and to issue identification cards and badges to them. If a traveler is victimized by a fake guide it is his own fault, for he should have insisted that the man show proper credentials.

In addition to its headquarters in Havana, the Tourist Commission has branches throughout Cuba, and offices in New York and Miami.

Chapter 49

GENERAL TRAVEL HINTS

UNITED STATES CITIZENS may visit Cuba without a passport. They should present documentary proof of some kind, such as a tax receipt or a driver's license, and in the case of naturalized citizens the immigration authorities may insist on seeing their final papers. But no hampering regulations are applied strictly to North Americans, unless there is reason to suspect the individual of being a criminal. Tourists of other countries must present their passports duly visaed for Cuba, along with return tickets, except that Canadian, French and in some circumstances British citizens are exempt from the visa.

When the traveler disembarks the transportation company gives him a blue tourist card, which is all he needs in the way of an identification paper. It is stamped by an

official and a small tax collected. This card must be surrendered on leaving the country; its loss would cause serious annoyance and delay.

Visitors are allowed to bring in, as part of their personal
baggage four hundred cigarettes, amateur cameras, portable
radios, and portable typewriters. The three last-mentioned
articles will be noted by the customs officer on the back of
the blue tourist card, and if the traveler does not have them
with him when he leaves he may be required to pay duty.

A tourist's automobile is allowed to enter Cuba free of
customs duty for a period 180 days (six months). Its own
license plates are good. If the passenger comes by plane,
he may have his car sent by ship and claim it as personal
baggage. It is even permissible to send from Cuba for the
car and to have it cleared on arrival as delayed baggage. A
temporary driving permit is issued without charge.

Foreign craft (sail, steam or motor power) and private
airplanes may come to Cuba with minimum formalities
and the payment of a few nominal fees.

A returning resident of the United States, provided he
has been abroad at least forty-eight hours, may take home
from Cuba $200 worth of purchases free of customs duty.
Only one hundred cigars and one gallon of alcoholic liquor
may figure in this exemption. After an absence from the
United States of longer than twelve days, the duty-free total
is increased by $200 or $300, depending on the circumstances. But additional cigars and liquor may not be included.

Local Transportation

Though legal rates have been fixed for Havana taxis,
there are no meters to control them. Special regulations
applying to zones and to night service make it difficult to
pin the driver down after the trip has been completed. It

is well therefore to bargain in advance for any trip that is
not routine. Be guided by the general schedule put out by
the Tourist Commission. Here are some standard charges:

Cab from the docks to downtown
  hotel,   1 to 3 persons, $1.00
Cab from Rancho Boyeros airport to
  any point in Havana,   1 to 3 persons, $4.00
Cab from Aerovias "Q" airport to any
  point in Havana,   1 to 3 persons, $2.50

Cuba has an efficient system of interurban buses. All the
lines leave and arrive now at the Omnibus Terminal, Rancho Boyeros highway, on the outskirts of the city. The
terminal has only lately been completed. It is a building
that offers every possible comfort, as well as varied shopping conveniences. In the main waiting room there is a
striking mural representing traffic, the central female figure
of which is by Armando Maribona.

The railroad system was started longer than a century
ago. A trunk line runs through the center of the island.
There are some branch lines, such as the one to Batabanó
on the south coast, and the independent Hershey electric
line which operates between Casa Blanca on the far side
of Havana harbor and the city of Matanzas. The main
railroad station in the capital is at Egido and Arsenal.

Planes serving the interior (Companía Cubana) use the
Rancho Boyeros airport, except that Aerovias "Q" which
offers daily flights to Varadero Beach and the Isle of Pines,
uses the airport at Columbia military camp, Marianao.

International plane service is for the most part through
Rancho Boyeros airport. A special autobus takes passengers
to the city for $1.00.

Steamer connections, which were disorganized by the

last World War and its aftermath, are now returning to normal. The P. & O.S.S. Co. has long maintained three sailings a week between Havana and Miami in the winter, and two a week in summer. Ships of the United Fruit Company and the Standard Fruit Company come to Havana weekly from New York and New Orleans, but instead of making the return trip direct they call first at Central American ports. The famous old Ward Line has resumed passenger activities with one sailing a week between Havana and New York.

The Companía Transatlantica Española has monthly sailings to Veracruz, Mexico, and to Spain via New York.

The Pacific Steam Navigation Company calls at Havana once every three months, en route from European ports to Jamaica and South America. Cars are accepted when the ship carries cargo for Kingston.

The Compagnie Générale Transatlantique (French Line) has resumed its service from Le Havre to Veracruz, via Havana.

Mail, Money, and Banks

Airmail to the United States, Canada, and Mexico costs eight cents per half ounce. To other Caribbean countries, including Central America, the charge is ten cents; to South America, fifteen cents and twenty cents; to Europe, twenty-five cents. Regular mail, first-class, within Cuba and to the United States is only two cents an ounce for letters and one cent for post cards; but there is talk of increasing the rate. Letter mail to all foreign countries except those of the Americas is at five cents an ounce.

The Cuban unit of currency is the peso, which has the same value as the United States dollar. The two are regarded as interchangeable in Havana, where even United States cents are accepted. The small coins issued locally are of values of one, two, five, ten, twenty and forty centavos. The twenty-centavo piece is called a peseta.

Cuban financial interests share the country's banking with powerful foreign institutions. The following are the chief houses in Havana: National City Bank of New York, Chase National Bank of the City of New York, First National Bank of Boston, Royal Bank of Canada, Bank of Nova Scotia, Trust Company of Cuba, and Banco del Comercio.

Periodicals

The three leading morning papers are *El Diario de la Marina*, *El Mundo* and *Información*. The first, founded in 1830, is the most conservative; it stresses the Iberian and Catholic viewpoint, and it tends to give too much of its space to society news. *El Mundo* and *Información* are livelier. Of the many afternoon papers in Spanish, *El País*, which puts out several editions, has the soundest reputation.

The Havana Post (morning) was launched more than fifty years ago during the American military occupation. It was for long the only English language paper in Cuba, and it is still the best.

Offsetting the fact that the afternoon dailies do not have Sunday editions, the morning papers do not publish on Monday.

In *Bohemia* and *Carteles* Havana has two illustrated weekly magazines which make a strong cultural appeal. *Bohemia*, in particular, is a leader among Latin American periodicals. Its ordinary editions usually exceed 100 pages, and it often issues specials that run to about 200 pages.

Chapter 50

TRIPS BEYOND THE SUBURBS

THIS IS a book about Havana, not one of travel in Cuba. However, there are a few trips to nearby points which practically every visitor makes, and it is logical to give some indications concerning them. Westward down the coast lies Mariel, just over the border of Pinar del Rio province. Due south from Havana is Batabanó on the Caribbean Sea. Eastward are (1) Guanabacoa, an inland point; (2) the Hershey sugar center and Jibacoa; (3) Varadero Beach, the most highly developed seashore resort in Cuba. So let us take them in that order.

Mariel, 36 miles from Havana, is on a beautiful small bay and is the site of Cuba's naval academy. The latter was founded in 1916. The castellated building which houses it originally belonged to Horatio Rubens, the North American lawyer who was a member of the Cuban junta in New York headed by José Martí. Rubens erected the structure for use as a casino, but never went ahead with this plan and disposed of his holding to the Cuban Government. The academy stands on a high bluff overlooking the village. On the point of land directly across the bay is the naval air base. If you tour the building and its annexes you will be pleased by the consistency of the architectural decorations, which all relate to the sea.

But many persons go to Mariel for the sake of the drive, the charm of the bay, and the delicious meals to be had at its two restaurants, the Villa Martin and the Hotel Miramar. I was first taken to Mariel twenty years ago by Conrado W. Massaguer, the caricaturist. We lunched on seafood just out of the water and listened to Spanish dance records by the great Encarnación López, "La Argentinita." Mariel has not changed. The trip is recommended to those who can be happy without meretricious excitement. On the way back it would be well to detour by Artemisa, a town in a beautiful landscape made singular by the extreme redness of the soil.

Batabanó, 35.5 miles from Havana, by way of the oldest route in western Cuba. The original site of Havana was on the south coast near Batabanó (see Chapter 2), and the settlers made their way north across the narrow waist of the island at this point. It is impossible to identify the location of the first settlement, but it was close to the modern town. The latter is not in itself attractive, apart from the Hotel Dos Hermanos where one eats well. The shallow waters of the bay, however, are of unfailing interest. The marine life of the bottom is visible for miles.

Sponge-reaping is the chief industry, though of late it has suffered from a disease that ruins the clustered growths. Experts peer down through glass-bottomed pails to identify the best sponges. There is also great activity in fishing, both for the market and for sport. Tarpon may be caught all the year round in the vicinity of Batabanó. Swordfish, pargo, pompano, wahoo, amber jack and all species of crustaceans are plentiful.

The roadstead (surgidero) lies about two miles beyond the town proper. Here you will find a long pier used by the steamer that maintains a service to the Isle of Pines, leaving Batabanó at 9:30 P.M. and arriving early in the morning.

Guanavacoa, within a few miles of the eastern outskirts of Havana. It can be reached by car or bus via several roads. The interest here rests in the township, which is extremely old. There was a Siboney village on the site before the coming of the Spaniards. Later the Crown tried to make it the concentration point of all surviving aboriginals in western Cuba, but it was too late to preserve the dying race.

Guanabacoa then became a fashionable settlement, where the best families of Havana built summer residences. Luckily many of the more beautiful houses are still in existence, including the palaces of the ennobled O'Reillys, the Casa Bayona, Prado Ameno, Villalba, and others. The streets on which they look are narrow, their doorways and grilled balconies are ornate. The parish church has a baroque high altar of considerable merit. In the convent of San Antonio, founded in 1755, the chapel and cloisters contain artistic woodwork. Guanabacoa as a whole is easily the finest relic of colonial days to be found within easy reach of the capital.

Hershey, twenty-eight miles by rail from Casa Blanca on the east side of Havana harbor. This is the sugar central of a North American company which has operated in Cuba for a generation or two. The trip is enjoyed by tourists because they are greeted in English and made to feel thoroughly at home. A good chance is afforded to see how sugar is manufactured from the cane and afterward refined. Most Cuban centrals ship their product raw to refineries abroad, but at Hershey's the entire process is completed. The company maintains a good, reasonably priced hotel, tennis courts, and a golf course, all of which are open to visitors. The new beach at Jibacoa is close by.

Varadero Beach, 114 miles from Havana by highway, thirty-five minutes by plane. It is also called the Playa

Azul (Blue Beach), not because the sands are tinted, but to describe the beauty of sea and sky so seldom clouded at that favored spot. Varadero is a development of the last thirty or thirty-five years. Its first enthusiast was the late Irénée Du Pont, the American munitions millionaire, who bought an estate because he was fascinated by the prospect of five miles of perfect white sand. The cleared stretch now is twelve miles. There are many hotels and private cottages.

Varadero is wonderful and every effort should be made to see it. Not everyone can afford to stay at its new Hotel Internacional, where the prices are staggering. But the pleasant old Casa La Rosa is still doing business, with a reasonable scale of charges, and there are other fairly modest resorts. Collectors of seashells will find Varadero rewarding, though in this respect it does not equal Baracoa at the far eastern end of Cuba. Above all, the visual effects will enchant North Americans, none of whose warm-water beaches can offer the background of rolling tropical terrain that marks Varadero.

INDEX